EQ-5D CONCEPTS AND METHODS

EQ-5D concepts and methods:
a developmental history

Edited by

PAUL KIND
University of York, U.K.

RICHARD BROOKS
University of Strathclyde, Strathclyde, Scotland

and

ROSALIND RABIN
EuroQol Group Business Management, The Netherlands

Springer

A C.I.P. Catalogue record for this book is available from the Library of Congress.

ISBN-10 1-4020-3711-2 (HB)
ISBN-10 1-4020-3712-0 (e-book)
ISBN-13 978-1-4020-3711-5 (HB)
ISBN-13 978-1-4020-3712-2 (e-book)

Published by Springer,
P.O. Box 17, 3300 AA Dordrecht, The Netherlands.

www.springeronline.com

Printed on acid-free paper

Printed in the Netherlands.

A collection of papers representing the collective
intellectual enterprise of the EuroQol Group

Presented to
Alan Williams

by his friends
in the EuroQol Group in Rotterdam,
October 1997

on the happy coincidence of his 70th birthday
and the 10th year of the Group's existence

Table of contents

List of contributors

Heleen van Agt, Department of Public Health, Erasmus Medical Center, Rotterdam, The Netherlands

Rikard Althin, Pfizer UK, Sandwich, Kent, United Kingdom

Xavier Badia, Health Outcomes Research Europe, Barcelona, Spain

Stefan Björk, Global Health Economics, Novo Nordisk A/S, Bagsvaerd, Denmark

Gouke Bonsel, Academic Medical Centre, Amsterdam, The Netherlands

Jan Busschbach, Institute for Medical Psychology & Psychotherapy, Erasmus Medical Center, Rotterdam, The Netherlands

Martin Buxton, Health Economics Research Group, Brunel University, London, United Kingdom

Frank de Charro, Centre for Health Policy and Law, Erasmus University Rotterdam, Rotterdam, The Netherlands

Paul Dolan, ScHARR, University of Sheffield, Sheffield, United Kingdom

Marie-Louise Essink-Bot, Department of Public Health, Erasmus Medical Center, Rotterdam, The Netherlands

Esteve Fernandez, Institut Català d'Oncologia (ICO), Barcelona, Spain

Julia Fox-Rushby, Health Economics Research Group, Brunel University, London, United Kingdom

Claire Gudex, Centre for Applied Health Services Research and Technology Assessment, University of Southern Denmark, Odense, Denmark

†Dick Hessing, Faculty of Law, Erasmus University Rotterdam, Rotterdam, The Netherlands

Ben van Hout, University Medical Centre, Utrecht, The Netherlands

Paul Kind, Outcomes Research Group, Centre for Health Economics, University of York, York, United Kingdom

Paul Krabbe, Department of Medical Technology Assessment, University Medical Centre Nijmegen, Nijmegen, The Netherlands

Joseph McDonnell, Institute for Medical Technology Assessment, Erasmus Medical Center, Rotterdam, The Netherlands

Erik Nord, Norwegian Institute of Public Health, Oslo, Norway

Ulf Persson, The Swedish Institute for Health Economics, Lund, Sweden

Arto Ohinmaa, Department of Public Health, University of Alberta, Edmonton, Canada

Rosalind Rabin, EuroQol Group Business Management, Rotterdam, The Netherlands

Montserrat Rue, Catalan Health Department, Lleida, Spain

†**Rachel Rosser**, Department of Psychiatry, University College London Medical School, London, United Kingdom

Andreu Segura, Institut d'Estudis de la Salut, Barcelona, Spain

Caroline Selai, Institute of Neurology, University College London, London, United Kingdom

Harri Sintonen, Department of Public Health, University of Helsinki, Helsinki, Finland

Alan Williams, Centre for Health Economics, University of York, York, United Kingdom

Foreword

Science today makes progress through the imaginative harvesting of knowledge generated by the many, rather than as the result of the isolated endeavours of the lone researcher. Innovations in the physical sciences from the development of nuclear technologies to the laser, have involved research teams working collectively. Collaboration is the rule rather than the exception. In the social sciences this model is all but reversed. Here it is not uncommon to encounter the solitary enthusiast, relishing an independence of spirit and pursuing their own private research agenda. All the more surprising then that a group of researchers from several different disciplines, should have come together in the late 1980s with nothing more substantial on the agenda than that they share their thoughts on the topic of measuring the value of health, or more specifically, on the way that the value of health might vary across different countries. Few scientific enterprises can have begun as cautiously or uncertainly. Few can have developed a cohesion and dynamism that lasted decades and continues to drive ahead after long years of scientific endeavour. Such is the good fortune that befell those of us who came together to form what was later to be known as the EuroQol Group. The Group's creation is principally due to the shared professional association of its members with one man, an economist by training and a visionary academic by inclination and temperament - Alan Williams. It was his catalytic influence that encouraged us all to participate in an initial exploratory session in Rotterdam in 1987. No one present had the remotest idea about the remarkable journey of discovery that lay ahead, or that a simple but effective health status measurement technology was to be the pay-off for the industry we undertook together.

The Group's founder members came from disparate disciplines and different environments - from health economics, medicine, sociology and psychology, from academia, health care, public health and government. Some, such as Rachel Rosser and Harri Sintonen, had already published their own independent measures of health status. From the outset they adopted a working practice based on openness and collegiality. All participants were credited with equal status. The way ahead lay through joint discussion of ideas and the formulation of methods for dealing with concepts and problems that obstructed progress. So as to explore the variation in values for health the Group needed a standard mechanism for describing health. Initially defined in terms of 6 dimensions, this classification was streamlined in 1993, taking on the form that is known today as EQ-5D. Since the Group was interested in exploring variation in values for health it logically followed that a standard valuation method was also required. Early on the Group adopted visual analogue scaling (VAS) utilizing a vertical 20cm scale calibrated, and sometimes referred to, as a "thermometer". A standard format was adopted too in regards to the design of a valuation questionnaire for use in postal surveys of the general population. The questionnaire elicited values for 16 health states presented in two groups of eight on separate pages. Health states were described as composites based on the standard descriptive system. Values for health states were indicated by drawing a line from the text box containing the health state description to the VAS "thermometer". Since both the concept of valuing health and the chosen technique for recording those values were likely to be foreign to most individuals presented with the task, it seemed obvious that some limited practice would be required. Two preliminary pages in the valuation questionnaire were designed to familiarize respondents with the descriptive system and the "thermometer" scale. It was only after early studies, designed to test practical issues of feasibility that it emerged that those two pages were capturing specific (and intriguing) information on respondent self-assessed health status. After much further experimentation[1] and some limited refinement, the current version of EQ-5D was published, following a 1993 moratorium on modification that has largely held until the present.

The reader is invited to sample this collection of research memorabilia with a degree of caution. Despite the dominant rationale of the EuroQol Group in developing the technology that now bears the label EQ-5D, the issues and themes to which it has given its attention speaks to a wider, more generalized audience. For the most part these issues are not in fact particular to EQ-5D, rather they are fundamental in nature and are expressed here as a local outcropping of a more substantial substrata. It must be recalled that, with the occasional exception, these papers were addressed to other members of the EuroQol Group as a contribution to a dynamic research agenda. There is therefore, an assumed level of knowledge that marks out these papers for a specialist audience. However, there is a high degree of transparency in their content so that the interested reader may easily transfer material into their own preferred area of competence. For those with a forensic inclination, the material contained within this volume might appear to offer some scope for exploitation. The EuroQol Group has a robust tradition of encouraging the free exchange of ideas and material amongst its members. It has never been the intention or practice to suppress well-informed criticism - quite the reverse. Group members are actively encouraged to confront the shortcomings of their own science. Hence it is possible to find those within the Group who advocate for, say, an increased number of response categories from 3 to 5, or that additional dimensions should be added to the standard 5. The Group has historically determined its position on such matters only after deliberating on the empirical evidence with which it is presented. Someone must generate that evidence and in so doing they need to break away from previously held positions, or the very least to test their robustness. Such incremental decision-making has only been only sustainable given the high quality research and the exercise of self-discipline that has been the hallmark of the Group for so long.

Despite the high standards aspired to by the EuroQol Group, there remain some aspects of its evolution that have proved to be an irritant in later years - starting with

---

1. Briefly summarized in Albrecht G L, Fitzpatrick R, editors. Advances in medical sociology : Quality of life in health care. JAI Press, 1994.

the name of the group itself. The founder members came from 4 countries (Finland, Netherlands, Sweden and the UK). They were concerned with measuring the value of health outcomes and since quality of life is heavily embedded in economic evaluation, it seemed natural at the time to refer in an almost casual way to the research network as the EuroQol Group. Continued usage led to the de facto labeling of that fraternity in precisely these terms. The term "EuroQol" for a while also (and unfortunately) became synonymous with the instrument designed to capture self-rated health status. Naming the component elements of what is now definitively termed EQ-5D was later the subject of some further difficult internal discussions. Had its founders only had the foresight to define and label in a standardized format then much of this could have been avoided. Thus the reader here will need to be aware that different authors may refer to the same components but using different terms. From an editorial perspective it might have been preferable to substitute EQ-5D for "The EuroQol Instrument" in the papers that form this volume. However, the intention in presenting this collection in their original format is to try and preserve the essential elements of the work using the language that was current within the Group at the time of writing.

The papers presented here span a 10-year period. They represent perhaps less than 10% of the total volume generated within the Group over that period and certainly less than 5% of its total output. The collection bears witness to the breadth of the developmental agenda that it tackled. They are rough diamonds, the unpolished source material that fuelled the evolutionary process. The papers map the developmental pathway that others have followed in pursuit of similar objectives. This collection specifically excludes more recent material since it was intended as a means of charting the Group's initial research product. From its formative steps, the EuroQol Group has evolved into a mature organization that continues to pursue its original research objective of investigating the valuation of health but combines this with a new role, as the corporate parent of EQ-5D. Were this volume to take account of more recent material, it could report that there are now more than 80 different language versions of EQ-5D and that soon a total of 2,000 studies will have been registered at the Group's website. The original group drew its members from amongst the research community in a handful of countries. Today that membership is global. The "Euro" in EuroQol was once mistakenly interpreted as indicating that EQ-5D was designed for local European users. Today its user base is worldwide. For those users who seek greater insights to the research work that underpins that status, this volume provides some documentary evidence.

The process of assembling such a volume was always going to be a challenge. The Group has produced a vast quantity of working papers. Its annual Scientific Plenary meetings now involve discussion of some 30 new texts each year. In the early days these meetings were twice as frequent but contained perhaps half the number of papers. Over the decade to 1997 there were literally hundreds of papers from which this selection was ultimately made. The cataloguing of this output has involved vari-

ous individuals, including Jan van Busschbach and Frank de Charro, given additional support by Erik Nord through the EuroQoLus system that he devised.
Much of the early material was never archived in electronic form and the physical preparation of these papers required significant input from Kerry Atkinson and Ben Kind in York. Further refinement and all pre-production was carried out in Rotterdam by Dennis Kennedy working with Rosalind Rabin. Richard Brooks has once again reentered the fray in his editorial role. Their collective input to the creation of this volume has been indispensable.

And finally, acknowledgement is due to the one individual in the Group who provided the inspiration and leadership in its formative days, wise counsel and sagacity in its adolescent years and who continues to stimulate new activity in what is now the approach of its 20th anniversary. To Alan Williams.

Paul Kind
Centre for Health Economics, University of York
April 2005

List of figures

1
The EuroQol Instrument

Alan Williams

The raison d'être of the EuroQol Instrument is to provide a simple "abstracting" device, for use alongside other more detailed measures of health-related quality of life (henceforth HRQoL), to serve as a basis for comparing health care outcomes using a basic "common core" of QoL characteristics which most people are known to value highly. From the outset it was accepted that for such comparisons to be useful it would be necessary to go beyond generating such information in the form of a "profile" (though the EuroQol data can be used in that way too), and therefore the issue of the relative valuation of different health states had to be confronted. It was further recognised that such information would be extremely valuable in a QALY-type context, but for that purpose it would be necessary to include a valuation for the state of being dead, otherwise it would be impossible to establish a cardinal index scale in which "dead" = 0 and "healthy" = 1, a property that is required for QALY-type calculations.

1.1 RESEARCH STRATEGY

People value both improvements in life expectancy and improvements in the quality of their lives, therefore any single index of the benefits of health care has to incorporate both. Ideally we would like to know how every individual values every possible prospective time profile of HRQoL, including the probabilities associated with each component in them. It need hardly be said that such an undertaking is impossible, so some strategic decisions have to be made concerning simplification of this research task. It is impossible to tell *a priori* which simplifications are best, so we are inevitably in the realm of intuition and scholarly judgement. It would therefore be most unwise for the research community to pursue only one strategy. What is called for is a broad range of different approaches, which need to be periodically reviewed to see what seems to be working and what does not.

1.2 THE DESCRIPTION OF HEALTH PROSPECTS

The particular simplifications involved in the approach adopted by the EuroQol Group were as follows:

(i) Each time profile of prospective health states is divided into separate time segments, such that within each segment the HRQoL of the individual is constant.

(ii) Initially it was to be assumed that the relative values attached to the different states were independent of the states that preceded or succeeded them, and of the length of time spent in each state.

P. Kind et al. (eds.), EQ-5D concepts and methods, 1–17.

Thus the Group rejected the scenario approach to health state description, in favour of using composite health states set out in a standardised manner. It was anticipated that at a later stage assumption (ii) could be relaxed, but in the meantime a common time duration was to be used (1 year), with the subject told that what happened thereafter was not known and should not be taken into account. The relaxation of this assumption is now under way within the Group, with data now becoming available from surveys undertaken in Finland and in The Netherlands. We too have experimental work about to start in the UK on the effect of varying the duration and the sequencing of states. Preliminary results are expected in October 1993.

A second set of simplifications is required concerning the detailed description of the health states themselves. There is an understandable tendency in this kind of enterprise to include everything that might be of any interest to anyone, and to work with fine enough gradations of "severity" within each "dimension" of HRQoL to pick up any effects of health care treatment that might be of interest to a discriminating practitioner. It is important here to recall that a 10-dimensional classification, with ten levels within each dimension, yields a classification system with 10^{10}, or 10000 million different cells. Such detail is quite inappropriate in an abstracting device, and if there is to be a reasonable prospect that such summary data is to be collected readily, it must be very simple to collect. If, for some other purpose, more detailed data is required it should be collected by an instrument designed for that specific purpose. Thus the general advice offered to prospective users is to use the (very simple) EuroQol Instrument alongside (not instead of) a more detailed specific measure, and, at this developmental stage in HRQoL measurement, preferably also alongside some more comprehensive generic measure (possibly one using the profile approach). This is now generating "calibration" data enabling systematic comparisons to be made between outcomes as measured by the EuroQol Instrument and outcomes as measured by other instruments.

The actual choice of descriptive content in the EuroQol Instrument originated from a review of existing instruments, the material so culled being reduced to manageable proportions through discussion between the original members of the Group, who ranged across many disciplines and who drew collectively on a wide range of experience. Later there was an opportunity to test these judgements against the results of a survey of lay concepts of health, which suggested that a dimension of "energy-tiredness" ought to be added to the original 6 dimensions. To accommodate this, 2 existing dimensions (1 concerned with work activities and the other with other activities) were fused, since it had transpired that the "other activities" dimension added little to the overall valuations of states. It turned out, however, that "energy/tiredness" also made little contribution to health state valuations, and in the pursuit of parsimony it was therefore dropped. This left us with the present 5-dimensional set, in which each dimension has 3 levels of "severity", generating 243 different cells (see Appendix 1.1). To these need to be added "unconscious" (because it cannot be regarded as a "composite" of the 5 dimensions) and "dead" (because it is required as a calibration point on the 0 to 1 scale), making 245 states in all.

1.3 THE VALUATION OF HEALTH PROSPECTS

Whilst in the process of establishing a workable descriptive system, the Group had also been devoting a great deal of attention to valuation issues. Early on it had been agreed that relative valuations should be sought for composite (multi-dimensional) states, not for each dimension separately. This important decision complicated the valuation task, because it involved rejection of the multi-attribute utility scaling approach, in case there proved to be significant interaction between the dimensions. But since no one subject could be expected to value more than a dozen or so states, this meant that the choice of states to be valued had to be made in such a way that, if necessary, it would be possible to estimate the values of all the other states from that limited number of observations. Thus a standard minimum set of (14) states was chosen which were to be used in all valuation work by all members, though where possible members were encouraged also to elicit values for a more extended set. From these states (plus a value for "being dead") the whole valuation space needs to be estimated. This is a task with which we are still experimenting with a variety of estimation techniques to see which uses our data most fully and produces the best fit.

For practical reasons the EuroQol Group imposed upon itself a very restrictive condition concerning the main body of data collection on relative valuations, namely that the questionnaire design should be so simple that it could be self-completed and conducted by a postal survey. This was essentially because none of us had research funds sizeable enough for any other alternative to be feasible, given that we wanted valuations from a general public, not from convenience samples. We quickly agreed that the only valuation method that would be practicable in that context was the visual analogue scale (VAS), and for this purpose we adopted a thermometer-like scale, the current form of which (see Appendix 1.1) is the result of considerable experimentation (using shorter, longer, differently calibrated, differently labelled, and differently orientated versions). The associated problem, which was also subjected to a fair amount of empirical testing, was the layout within the questionnaire of the states to be valued. A complication here was that in order to standardise "framing" effects we had to repeat some states on subsequent pages, thereby reducing the number of observations available to us. But the most difficult issue with the visual analogue scale has been getting people to value the state of "being dead" alongside the other states, and this is still an active area of experimentation within the Group.

Lately, with more research funds being devoted to this kind of research, it has been possible to generate valuations for EuroQol states using valuation methods other than the VAS, and in particular comparing those valuations with ones derived from the Standard-Gamble (SG) and the Time-Trade-Off (TTO) methods. From preliminary work, there appears to be a power- function relationship between the VAS and each of the other 2 methods. It further appears that the TTO method yields somewhat better quality data than the SG method, if quality is judged by the internal consistency of the answers given by respondents, the sensitivity of valuations to parameters known to influence them, and the reliability of the responses when the valuation task is repeated by the same respondents some weeks later. For this reason the TTO method will be used alongside the VAS (thermometer) in the next round of our own work, which is now under way.

This next round of work is to consist of just over 3000 interviews with a representative sample of the adult population of the UK living in their own homes. Valuations will be sought on about 40 EuroQol states, carefully selected so as to be well spread through the valuation space, and to be particularly useful for the estimation of the values of the states on which we shall have no direct valuations. Respondents will each value a stratified random sample of 15 of these 40 or so states, using first a simple ranking of states, then a rating on the "thermometer" (using the method of "bisection", so as to generate an interval scale), and finally the TTO method. The fieldwork is being conducted with Social and Community Planning and Research (SCPR), who have worked with us over the past year or so to develop this interview-based format. We anticipate that the fieldwork will be completed by the end of 1993, and the preliminary results available around Easter 1994. We hope to be able to deliver a full report to the Health Economics Study Group (HESG) at the Summer Meeting in 1994. At that point we expect to have a tariff of values for all EuroQol states which will be representative of the views of the UK public. We are at the very early stages of developing a parallel study to elicit the values of doctors and nurses by identical methods, to see how they compare with each other, and with the views of the general public.

A widespread concern with all HRQoL measurement is the validity and reliability of each particular measure. In general, establishing "validity" requires the investigator to address the question "does your measure measure what it purports to measure?". But since there is no "gold standard" for the measurement of health-related quality of life, this seems an unanswerable question. So what people fall back on instead are appeals to plausibility, for instance: testing whether the measure contains the kind of elements that we would expect such a measure to have; whether it goes up when we would expect it to go up and down when we would expect it to go down; and so on. These are all very subjective notions, and ultimately rely heavily on intuition and professional judgement. We know from our own earlier work:

(i) that EuroQol self-rated health on the VAS thermometer declines (as expected) with age, and
(ii) that whilst self-reported pain and discomfort increase with age, anxiety and depression decrease with age, and
(iii) that people's valuations are affected both by age and by experience of illness.

My own personal view is that searching for "validity" in this field, at this stage in the history of HRQoL measurement, is like chasing a will o' the wisp, and probably equally unproductive. It would, however, be useful to find out whether the values elicited from particular individuals in particular circumstances are consistent with their actual behaviour when they are put in a situation in which those values should have been crucial. The devising, conduct and interpretation of the results of such a study would be a valuable contribution to this otherwise rather murky area.

Reliability refers to the issue as to whether the values elicited from an individual are stable, which is usually tested by (surreptitiously?) repeating a question at different stages within an interview, or by going back to the individual a short while later in order to see whether on the second occasion the same answers are obtained as on the first occasion. Within the context of a short self-completed questionnaire the former method does not seem appropriate, and if (as they usually are) questionnaires are returned anonymously, the latter method is not possible. But in recent interviewer-led survey work we have been able to use the latter method, and it appears that the valuations elicited in that context are stable and reliable.

1.4 THE EUROQOL INSTRUMENT AND THE MEASUREMENT OF QUALITY OF LIFE

The EuroQol Instrument has two distinct contributions to make to the task of measuring health-related quality of life. First, it offers a very convenient way of collecting descriptive data about HRQoL, and about people's own self-rating of their current health state (by using only pages 2 and 3 of the questionnaire in Appendix 1.1). This descriptive data is needed if we are to fill the gaps in our knowledge about the HRQoL sequelae of many common health care activities. The second, and much more ambitious, role is that of supplying a tariff of social values of health states, to be used (alongside cost data) in a planning context when determining priorities for health care. Each of these distinct, but related, roles will now be considered in turn.

1.5 THE DESCRIPTIVE ROLE

Concerning the descriptive role of the data which can be collected using *only* pages 2 and 3 of the EuroQol questionnaire, this produces (from page 2) a simple description by patients of their health-related quality of life. This requires only that five ticks are entered on to the form, which is essentially just page 2 of Appendix 1.1.

It takes less than a minute to complete, and can either be self-assessed or observer-assessed. The data can be summarised, in profile form, as a simple 5-digit code. There are, however, considerable advantages in going beyond this stage and adding the self-rating exercise shown on page 3 of Appendix 1.1. These additional data enable a single summary statistic to be generated, which can either be used in conjunction with the 5-digit code, or as a measure of self-rated health in its own right. It may be analysed either in a cross-sectional manner when pooled with similar data from other subjects, or it may be used in a longitudinal manner to trace out each individual's rating of own health at different points in time. It is probably more safely used in the latter manner than in the former, since optimistic people may rate all states higher than pessimistic people do, but each will rate the direction of change in their health accurately.

As was indicated earlier, the EuroQol Instrument was not designed as a "stand alone" instrument for measuring all kinds of HRQoL in sufficient detail for all purposes. It was designed as an "abstracting" device, to be used alongside other measures as necessary, and intended to provide information about a common core of key items, which should always be of interest, because they represent people's salient concerns about HQQoL. Because of its summary, generic nature, it is likely that it will normally be used alongside other more detailed measures, either of a generic or of a specific nature, which focus on the particular concerns of the investigators in each study.

This opens up the possibility of systematic within-subject comparison of the EuroQol descriptions with the descriptions generated by other methods. This would enable these other descriptions to be given a EuroQol score, using our tariff. Where the other methods also generate a single summary score, it also opens up the possibility of recalibrating these other scores using the EuroQol valuations. Once sufficient data of this comparative kind were available, it should be possible to attach EuroQol scores directly to data which was collected solely with other instruments. Where the alternative instrument is a generic instrument (such as the Nottingham Health Profile (NHP) or Short Form 36 (SF-36)) it should be possible to establish a fairly close mapping of the more detailed instrument onto the simpler EuroQol system. It may be more difficult with disease-specific or treatment-specific measures, since they will typically not cover such a broad range of dimensions as a generic measure, concentrating on depth rather than breadth of coverage.

There are, therefore, limitations to this enterprise. One is that, even where a broad range of HRQoL dimensions is tracked by other instruments, they are not usually reported in sufficient detail for this recalibration to be possible. To move from a series of frequency distributions relating to a group of patients in a trial, to the particular combination of characteristics manifested by individual subjects, requires quite sweeping assumptions about the interrelationships between the different elements which may be difficult to sustain. This means that it may be necessary to engage in the delicate and time-consuming business of persuading researchers to give access to their primary data for the purposes of secondary analysis, a process fraught with personal, professional and practical difficulties. A second major limitation arises when the other measure used alongside the EuroQol measure is limited to a narrow range of dimensions (e.g. if it is concerned only with mood, or only with mobility). In such cases we have no information whatever about where a patient stands on the other EuroQol dimensions, and if all we can elicit from the specific measure is that (say) the person is moderately depressed, all we could record within the EuroQol descriptive system is the 5-digit code "****2" (* indicating that the other digits are unknown). In this situation, the range of possible EuroQol states into which the patient might fall is enormous (there are 81 of them!), and so therefore is the range of possible valuations attached to the rather cryptic state "****2".

Fraught with difficulties though it may be, this is nevertheless an activity which must be pursued. Preliminary work of this kind is already in hand comparing EuroQol with SF-36 and the NHP, and we have already persuaded about 30 investigators to use the EuroQol Instrument within their studies, usually alongside other instruments. Here it is important to distinguish between two different kinds of HRQoL measure; those whose weights are derived from people's preferences or values, and those whose weights are derived in some other way (e.g. for their predictive power). The SF-36 is of the latter variety, and so it is especially important to map it onto a measure with preference weights. In the case of the NHP, the weights within each of the 6 dimensions were generated by eliciting people's preferences, but different people were consulted for each dimension, and no preferences across dimensions were elicited. Since the EuroQol method presents composite health states for relative valuation, it fills a void in the NHP system of generating weights.

1.6 THE QALY ROLE

For the purpose of QALY calculation the descriptive material generated on page 2 of the EuroQol Instrument needs to have applied to it a tariff representing the social valuation of the state in question, and this is the role our 1994 tariff is intended to fulfil. An additional concern is frequently voiced here, namely how can we be sure that we have generated a scale with the required interval properties?

It has been argued by one member of the EuroQol Group that the use of the visual analogue scale tends to compress valuations at one end of the scale (Nord, 1991). On the other hand it appears that if the EuroQol data is treated purely as ordinal, and analysed as pairwise comparisons using a measurement model (e.g. Thurstone's) which is known to generate an interval scale, it yields a scale which is very close to the scale obtained when the VAS data is interpreted as cardinal data (Kind, Personal Communication, 1993). We are hoping that the use of the "bisection" method with the rating scale in our current survey work will help to resolve this issue.

1.7 ONGOING TASKS

The EuroQol Instrument is in a continual state of development and further experimentation, and we welcome collaboration from others who are willing to pursue any of the developmental tasks in which they are interested and which they have the resources to undertake. In particular we are at present seeking collaboration with people helping to set up evaluative studies which are using any HRQoL measures, so as to get pages 2 and 3 of the EuroQol Instrument used alongside whatever other measures are in use. This will greatly facilitate the "calibration" exercise mentioned earlier.

But this "calibration" has a much deeper significance in relation to the development of QALY League Tables. Those currently in existence have been criticised (Gerard and Mooney, 1993; Drummond *et al*, 1993) because neither the benefit measures nor the cost measures are sufficiently standardised to ensure that the comparisons are valid. On the benefit side this is precisely the task that the EuroQol Instrument was designed to tackle, and it must be a strong contender for that "common core" role. Moreover, because it separates description from valuation, and has a standard system for generating valuations which can be applied to different target populations, it means that "local" valuations (i.e. those from a particular subset of the population) could be used if these differ from "national" valuations (in our 1994 tariff we may even be able to generate different tariffs for different subsets of the population for use where such a differential tariff is considered appropriate). The sooner we get on with the collection of this comparative descriptive data, the sooner will we be able to produce better comparisons of relative outcomes from different interventions, which is a key element in the use of "health gain" in priority setting in health care.

Originally presented to the Health Economists Study Group, Strathclyde, Scotland, 1993

1.8 REFERENCES

Drummond M, Torrance G, Mason J. Cost-effectiveness league tables - more harm than good. Soc Sci & Med 1993;37(1):33-40.

Gerard K, Mooney G. QALY league tables: handle with care. Health Econ. 1993;2(1):59-64.

Nord E. The validity of a visual analogue scale in determining social utility weights for health states. Int J of Health Planning and Management 1991;6:234-242.

APPENDIX 1.1

THE EQ-5D VALUATION QUESTIONNAIRE (INCLUDES EQ-5D)

Health Questionnaire

We are trying to find out what people think about health. We are going to describe a few health states that people can be in. We want you to indicate how good or bad each of these states would be for a person like you. There are no right or wrong answers. Here we are interested only in your personal view.

But first of all we would like you to indicate (on the next page) the state of your own health today.

By placing a tick in one box in each group below, please indicate which statements best describe your own health state today.

Mobility
I have no problems in walking about ☐
I have some problems in walking about ☐
I am confined to bed ☐

Self-Care
I have no problems with self-care ☐
I have some problems washing or dressing myself ☐
I am unable to wash or dress myself ☐

Usual Activities *(e.g. work, study, housework, family or leisure activities)*
I have no problems with performing my usual activities ☐
I have some problems with performing my usual activities ☐
I am unable to perform my usual activities ☐

Pain/Discomfort
I have no pain or discomfort ☐
I have moderate pain or discomfort ☐
I have extreme pain or discomfort ☐

Anxiety/Depression
I am not anxious or depressed ☐
I am moderately anxious or depressed ☐
I am extremely anxious or depressed ☐

To help people say how good or bad a health state is, we have drawn a scale (rather like a thermometer) on which the best state you can imagine is marked 100 and the worst state you can imagine is marked 0.

We would like you to indicate on this scale how good or bad your own health is today, in your opinion. Please do this by drawing a line from the box below to whichever point on the scale indicates how good or bad your health state is today.

Your own health state today

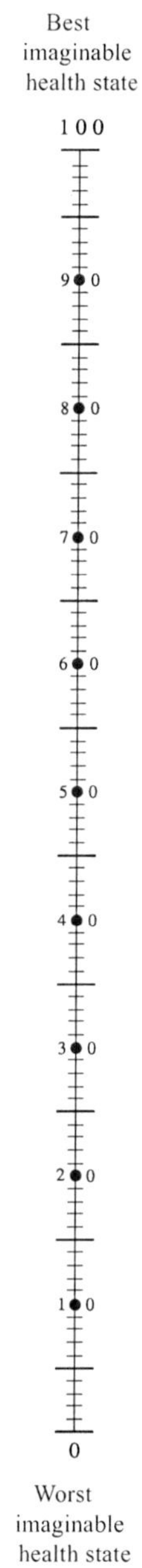

- We now want you to consider some other health states.

- Remember, we want you to indicate how good or bad each of these states would be for a person like you.

- They are described, on either side of the scale, on the page opposite.

- When thinking about each health state imagine that it will last for one year. What happens after that is not known and should not be taken into account.

- Please draw **one line from each box** to whichever point on the scale indicates how good or bad the state described in that box is.

- It does not matter if your lines cross each other.

Best
imaginable
health state

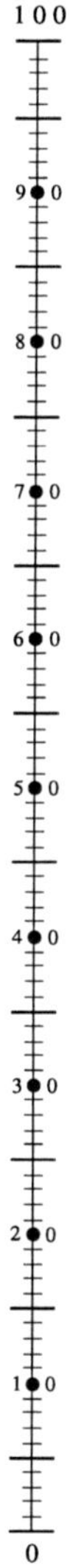

No problems in walking about
No problems with self-care
Some problems with performing usual activities *(e.g. work, study, housework, family or leisure activities)*
No pain or discomfort
Not anxious or depressed

No problems in walking about
No problems with self-care
No problems with performing usual activities *(e.g. work, study, housework, family or leisure activities)*
Moderate pain or discomfort
Not anxious or depressed

No problems in walking about
No problems with self-care
No problems with performing usual activities *(e.g. work, study, housework, family or leisure activities)*
No pain or discomfort
Not anxious or depressed

Some problems in walking about
Some problems with washing or dressing self
Some problems with performing usual activities *(e.g. work, study, housework, family or leisure activities)*
Extreme pain or discomfort
Extremely anxious or depressed

Some problems in walking about
No problems with self-care
Some problems with performing usual activities *(e.g. work, study, housework, family or leisure activities)*
Extreme pain or discomfort
Moderately anxious or depressed

Confined to bed
Unable to wash or dress self
Unable to perform usual activities *(e.g. work, study, housework, family or leisure activities)*
Extreme pain or discomfort
Extremely anxious or depressed

No problems in walking about
No problems with self-care
No problems with performing usual activities *(e.g. work, study, housework, family or leisure activities)*
Moderate pain or discomfort
Moderately anxious or depressed

Confined to bed
Unable to wash or dress self
Unable to perform usual activities *(e.g. work, study, housework, family or leisure activities)*
Moderate pain or discomfort
Not anxious or depressed

Worst
imaginable
health state

PLEASE CHECK THAT YOU HAVE DRAWN ONE LINE FROM EACH BOX (THAT IS, 8 LINES IN ALL)

5

IN THE SAME WAY AS ON THE PREVIOUS PAGE, PLEASE INDICATE HOW GOOD OR BAD THESE ADDITIONAL STATES ARE, BY DRAWING A LINE FROM EACH BOX TO A POINT ON THE SCALE.

YOU WILL FIND THAT 2 OF THESE STATES (MARKED *) ARE REPEATED FROM THE PREVIOUS PAGE.

Best imaginable health state

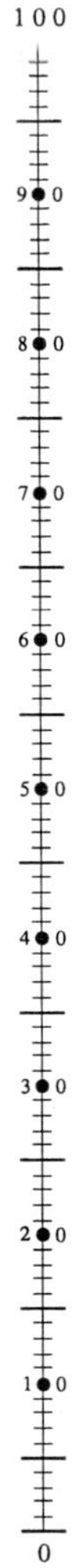

Worst imaginable health state

Some problems in walking about
No problems with self-care
No problems with performing usual activities *(e.g. work, study, housework, family or leisure activities)*
No pain or discomfort
Not anxious or depressed

No problems in walking about
No problems with self-care
No problems with performing usual activities *(e.g. work, study, housework, family or leisure activities)*
No pain or discomfort
Moderately anxious or depressed

No problems in walking about *
No problems with self-care
No problems with performing usual activities *(e.g. work, study, housework, family or leisure activities)*
No pain or discomfort
Not anxious or depressed

Confined to bed
Some problems with washing or dressing self
Some problems with performing usual activities *(e.g. work, study, housework, family or leisure activities)*
No pain or discomfort
Not anxious or depressed

Unconscious

Confined to bed *
Unable to wash or dress self
Unable to perform usual activities *(e.g. work, study, housework, family or leisure activities)*
Extreme pain or discomfort
Extremely anxious or depressed

No problems in walking about
Some problems with washing or dressing self
No problems with performing usual activities *(e.g. work, study, housework, family or leisure activities)*
No pain or discomfort
Not anxious or depressed

Some problems in walking about
Some problems with washing or dressing self
Unable to perform usual activities *(e.g. work, study, housework, family or leisure activities)*
Moderate pain or discomfort
Extremely anxious or depressed

PLEASE CHECK THAT YOU HAVE DRAWN ONE LINE FROM EACH BOX (THAT IS, 8 LINES IN ALL)

6

- In the previous pages we asked you to say how good or bad various health states are in your view.

- We would now like you to tell us how good or bad you feel the state 'dead' is, compared with being in the other states for one year.

- Please turn back to pages 5 **and** 6 and draw one line across the thermometer at the point you would locate the state 'dead'.

- Remember we would like you to do this on **both** pages 5 and 6.

Because all replies are anonymous, it will help us to understand your answers better if we have a little background data from everyone, as covered in the following questions. (At the end there is space to add anything else you think may be helpful to us).

	Yes	No	
1. Have you experienced serious illness?			PLEASE TICK APPROPRIATE BOXES
in you yourself	☐	☐	
in your family	☐	☐	
in caring for others	☐	☐	

2. What is your age in years? ☐

	Male	Female	
3. Are you:	☐	☐	PLEASE TICK APPROPRIATE BOX

4. Are you: (PLEASE TICK APPROPRIATE BOX)
   - *a current smoker* ☐
   - *an ex-smoker* ☐
   - *a never smoker* ☐

	Yes	No	
5. Do you now, or did you ever, work in health or social services?	☐	☐	PLEASE TICK APPROPRIATE BOX

If so, in what capacity? ☐

6. Which of the following best describes your main activity? (PLEASE TICK APPROPRIATE BOX)
   - *in employment or self employment* ☐
   - *retired* ☐
   - *housework* ☐
   - *student* ☐
   - *seeking work* ☐
   - *other (please specify)* ☐ ☐

	Yes	No	
7. Did your education continue after the minimum school leaving age?	☐	☐	PLEASE TICK APPROPRIATE BOX
8. Do you have a Degree or equivalent professional qualification?	☐	☐	PLEASE TICK APPROPRIATE BOX

9. Please add here any comments you may wish to make which might help us to understand your answers better:

10. Did you find filling in this questionnaire:

very difficult	☐	PLEASE TICK APPROPRIATE BOX
fairly difficult	☐	
fairly easy	☐	
very easy	☐	

11. Could you please let us know roughly how long it took you to complete (in minutes): ☐

12. If you know your postcode, would you please write it here: ☐

Thank you for being so helpful

2
The descriptive system of the EuroQol Instrument

Claire Gudex

2.1 OBJECTIVES

In determining the coverage and structure of the EuroQol descriptive system, it was important to keep in mind the objectives of the instrument itself. Thus the EuroQol was to be a generic instrument for describing and valuing health-related quality of life (HRQoL), providing both a descriptive profile and an overall index for HRQoL. While it should be capable of identifying differences between populations and population groups, it was not intended to be a comprehensive measure of HRQoL, but as a standardised tool to facilitate the collection of a common data set. The instrument was also intended to be self-completed, and to be acceptable for use in postal surveys.

The concept of HRQoL used was broadly in line with the definition later suggested by Patrick and Erickson, 1993 - 'the value assigned to duration of life as modified by the impairments, functional states, perceptions and social opportunities that are influenced by disease, injury, treatment or policy'. The dimensions chosen should aim to capture physical, mental and social functioning, as the basic elements of relevance to a generic measure (Brooks, 1995). It should be noted that the development of the EuroQol took place mainly in northern Europe, with an inevitable bias towards cultural concepts appropriate to that part of the world. However, a recent population survey conducted in Spain suggests that the descriptive system is applicable there (Badia *et al,* 1995). No formal testing has been conducted in non-western cultures, although experimental studies in eastern Europe, Thailand, and among Bangladeshis living in England have been successful.

The objectives of the EuroQol enterprise led to certain requirements for the descriptive system. Firstly, in order to generate a generic instrument, the dimensions should be relevant to patients across the spectrum of health care, as well as to members of the general population. Thus there would be no mention of specific diagnoses, diseases or treatments, while disease-specific items, such as symptoms, would not be included. Such a demarcation is not always clear, in that a feeling of depression can be a symptom or a diagnosis in itself. However, the criterion for a dimension was that, even though it may figure largely in a particular illness or disease, it should also be of relevance to a wide range of patients and to the general population.

Secondly, the descriptive system should be fairly simple in order to generate a feasible number of potential health states for valuation purposes. In this respect the EuroQol Group has been motivated by an important strategic consideration. Within the

P. Kind et al. (eds.), EQ-5D concepts and methods, 19–27.

field of HRQoL measurement, there are two different, and to some extent opposing, schools of thought. While both agree that HRQoL is a multidimensional phenomenon, the first believes that this should be preserved at all costs and that HRQoL can only be represented as a profile of scores ascross discrete dimensions. The EuroQol Group is, however, grounded in the second school, which believes that health status can be modelled on a unidimensional continuum that permits point observations to be represented by a single index score. Furthermore, rather than weighting each dimension separately and then using some sort of additive or multiplicative process to combine them, it was desired to value whole health states so that the resulting valuations would incorporate interactions between dimensions. Thus, not only could changes in 1 dimension be detected (as with a profile measure), but when there was an improvement on 1 dimension and a deterioration on another, this information could be reconciled to produce a measure of net subjective change across all dimensions.

This valuation approach requires respondents to value whole health states and, ideally, for each respondent to value as many states as possible, if not all potential health states. The descriptive system therefore needs to be simple, using as few dimensions as possible, and as few items as possible within each dimension. The number of potential health states grows rapidly with an increase in the number of items or dimensions e.g. an instrument with 2 items in each of 3 dimensions generates 8 (2^3) health states, while one with 6 dimensions, each with 4 items, generates 4096 (4^6) states. As a further consideration, the description of a health state needs to be fairly short and sufficiently clear so that the respondent can identify differences between the states, particularly those that may differ by only 1 item. It was therefore considered preferable to present the items within each health state as bullet points rather than in a more narrative style.

The final requirement was that the instrument should be amenable to self-completion in a range of settings e.g. in a busy hospital clinic or in the respondent's own home. The instrument should be simple enough not to require detailed instructions, and the descriptive page should only take a couple of minutes to complete. A small number of dimensions and items, with an easy response form was therefore desirable. It was considered that placing a tick or a cross in the appropriate boxes was the most usual and straightforward way for respondents to answer.

2.2 SELECTION OF DIMENSIONS

It was evident from the beginning that a compromise had to be made between the desire to have a comprehensive instrument covering all the dimensions that other HRQol instruments had used, and the need for a simple instrument that would be feasible in practice. A selection process was needed to choose from the large number of potential dimensions. The Group discussed various alternatives, including a survey of patients and the general population to identify common dimensions of relevance to all groups. From the large amount of data produced, it would then be possible to identify such dimensions, although the ultimate choice would be heavily influenced by the expectations and biases of the researchers - there would still need to be some value judgement about which of the many 'important' dimensions should be included. In acknowledging this subjectivity in the choice of descriptive dimensions, the EuroQol Group decided to take an alternative strategy, by drawing on their own expertise to select the dimensions.

The Group undertook a detailed review of other generic HRQoL measures available at the time. These included the Quality of Well-Being (Patrick *et al,* 1973), the Sickness Impact Profile (Bergner *et al,* 1976), the Nottingham Health Profile (Hunt and McEwen, 1980), the Rosser Index (Rosser and Kind, 1978), the Health Measurement Questionnaire (Kind and Gudex, 1991) and the 15-D (Sintonen, 1981).

Contrary to expectations, the dimensions suggested for inclusion by the various members of the Group were broadly similar, with differences relating more to the names of dimensions rather than to their contents. There was general agreement that the following dimensions should be included in a basic HRQoL tool: mobility, daily activities and self-care, psychological functioning, social and role performance, and pain or other health problems.

2.3 SELECTION OF ITEMS

Items were chosen so as to be of ordinal character within each dimension, and to cover a wide range of severity within each dimension. Thus there should be scope for application in many different settings and populations, from healthy people living in their own homes and going about their usual activities, to severely ill patients in hospital. Thus the first item was always 'no problem', while the last item was the most extreme possible answer e.g. 'extreme pain, unable to do'. Where there was a third level, this was intended to be roughly in the middle of the continuum between 'no problem' and 'extreme problem'.

A consequence of developing the instrument within a multidisciplinary and multi-lingual group was that considerable importance was placed on identifying words that conveyed a similar meaning to people with different backgrounds and from different cultures. Indeed, there were many words suggested in one language that could not be translated sufficiently closely into another language. The great benefit of this exercise taking place round a table was that the meaning and wording of each dimension could be discussed, and we were able to reach a general consensus over the interpretation of the dimension. Simultaneous translation ensured that both the dimension and its items were likely to be readily understood in the national setting.

Care was also taken to avoid medical or technical terminology, preferring everyday usual language. Where uncertainties remained, it was possible to conduct a short survey to test the effects of using different words e.g. the use of 'strong pain' rather than 'extreme pain' in the Norwegian version.

2.4 THE EUROQOL 6D DESCRIPTIVE SYSTEM

The descriptive system that emerged in 1988 from the review of other generic measures consisted of 6 dimensions, each with either 2 or 3 items (Table 2.1). A person's health state was described as a 6-figure number, by selecting one item (coded 1, 2 or 3) from each dimension e.g. state 212221 meant problems in walking but no problems with self-care, inability to perform work or leisure activities, moderate pain or discomfort but no anxiety or depression. Theoretically, this set of dimensions and items generated 216 (2^3 x 3^3) permutations. Physical functioning was encompassed in the 'mobility' and 'self-care' dimensions, social functioning in the 'social relationships' dimension, and mental functioning in the 'anxiety/depression' dimension.

Table 2.1 Original 6D EuroQol descriptive system

Mobility	
1.	No problems walking about
2.	Unable to walk about without a stick, crutch or walking frame
3.	Confined to bed
Self-care	
1.	No problems with self-care
2.	Unable to dress self
3.	Unable to feed self
Main activity	
1.	Able to perform main activity (e.g. work, study, housework)
2.	Unable to perform usual activity
Social relationships	
1.	Able to pursue family and leisure activities
2.	Unable to pursue family and leisure activities
Pain	
1.	No pain or discomfort
2.	Moderate pain or discomfort
3.	Extreme pain or discomfort
Mood	
1.	Not anxious or depressed
2.	Anxious or depressed

There was considerable discussion of the implications of having a dichotomous dimension, such as pain/discomfort or anxiety/depression. It was acknowledged that this might cause ambiguity for respondents, but the alternative of making each dimension separate had too large an implication for the potential number of health states.

Following a large national survey of lay concepts of health (van Dalen *et al*, 1994), an investigaton was conducted as to whether an additional dimension of energy/tiredness should be incorporated into the EuroQol classification. The results of the survey had suggested that the EuroQol descriptive system sufficiently covered the dimensions of particular importance to people, except for the frequently mentioned one of energy/vitality. However, the inclusion of an energy/tiredness dimension into the 6D schema was found to have no significant effects either on self-reported health or on the valuation of other health states, and regression analysis showed no clear contribution from an energy dimension (Gudex, 1992). The extra dimension was thus not incorporated into the EuroQol descriptive system.

2.5 THE EUROQOL 5D DESCRIPTIVE SYSTEM

In the light of initial experiments with the 6D version, a number of changes were made, resulting in a descriptive system with 5 dimensions, each with 3 items (Table 2.2). This version was formally ratified by the Group in 1990.

It was considered that each dimension should have the same number of items, providing a more balanced structure to the descriptive system, and giving equal importance to each item in the resulting composite health states. In addition, semantic changes were made in order to create the same structure within each dimension i.e. 'no' problems, 'some or moderate' problems, and 'unable or extreme' problems. Under the mobility dimension, the second level was further changed so as to not exclude people who used other types of walking aid, or people who had problems walking but did not use an aid.

Table 2.2 5D EuroQol descriptive system

Mobility

1. No problems in walking about
2. Some problems in walking about
3. Confined to bed

Self-care

1. No problems with self-care
2. Some problems washing or dressing self
3. Unable to wash or dress self

Usual activities

1. No problems with performing usual activities
   (e.g. work, study, housework, family or leisure activities)
2. Some problems with performing usual activities
3. Unable to perform usual activities

Pain/Discomfort

1. No pain or discomfort
2. Moderate pain or discomfort
3. Extreme pain or discomfort

Anxiety/Depression

1. Not anxious or depressed
2. Moderately anxious or depressed
3. Extremely anxious or depressed

Note: For convenience each composite health state has a 5 digit code number relating to the relevant level of each dimension, with the dimensions always listed in the order given above. Thus 11232 means:

1 No problems walking about

1 No problems with self-care

2 Some problems with performing usual activities

3 Extreme pain or discomfort

2 Moderately anxious or depressed

A major change was made to the dimension of self-care. The third item, relating to inability to feed oneself, was marked by very few respondents and was felt to be too specific for use in most patient groups. The ability to wash oneself was agreed to be more relevant, and was thus included along with dressing oneself.

Adding an extra dimension to 3 of the dimensions (main activity, social relationships and mood) had severe consequences for the number of potential health states described by the system. A total of 729 (3^6) states were then described, and this was felt to be too large a number for the later valuation task. It was finally agreed to take out 'social relationships' as a separate dimension as it had been shown to contribute little to the valuation of health states. It was subsumed under what was previously the 'main activity' dimension, which was changed to explicitly mention family and leisure activities alongside work, study and housework.

2.6 VALIDITY OF THE DESCRIPTIVE SYSTEM

The descriptive system is presented to respondents on page 2 of the EuroQol Instrument. It can be used to indicate whether a respondent has a problem on any of the dimensions, and, if so, how severe this problem is. The same data from a number of individuals can be aggregated to obtain a descriptive HRQoL profile for a particular patient or population group. As a further step, a score can be given to each health state so described, either by asking respondents themselves to rate their own health, or by applying a score from a social tariff (see later chapters).

In view of the objectives of the EuroQol Instrument, the performance of the descriptive system can be assessed in a variety of ways. Does it include all the necessary dimensions for a generic, common core instrument of HRQoL i.e. does it have content validity? Does it produce results concordant with those from other HRQoL instruments or related measures i.e. does it have convergent validity? For example does a respondent scoring poorly on mobility on the EuroQol also score poorly on physical mobility on the SF-36? Is a relationship between status and age identified, where older respondents might be expected to report more problems with mobility and self-care than younger respondents? Does it identify differences that would be expected between respondent groups i.e. does it have discriminant validity? For example, patients with arthritis would be expected to indicate more problems on mobility and greater pain than others of a similar age in the general population, while people with acute asthma might be expected to report more problems with performing usual activities and a greater degree of anxiety or depression. Does the descriptive system identify changes across time i.e. does it show sensitivity to change? Being a simple generic system, it is unlikely to identify small differences across time (these may instead be identified through the use of self-rated own health on page 3 of the instrument), but it should still be capable of recognising clinically important changes - particularly as the descriptive system is intended as the basis for applying scores from a social tariff.

2.7 SUMMARY

The EuroQol descriptive system has developed within the context of a generic, index measure of HRQoL. Dimensions have been chosen based on a conceptual process rather than by statistical means such as factor analysis, and have been identified through a review of other generic health status measures. Emphasis has been placed on identifying a common core set of dimensions rather than attempting comprehensive coverage of all those possible, allowing the instrument to be used alongside both other generic measures as well as disease-specific instruments. Another strategic consideration was the requirement to generate a feasible number of health states for later valuation.

The result is a 5-dimensional system covering mobility, self-care, usual activities, pain/discomfort and anxiety/depression. With 3 levels within each dimension, a total of 243 different health states are described. This system can be used to generate a profile of HRQoL for a single individual, a group of patients, or a whole population, and can also be used to assess changes in HRQoL across time.

Presented at the EuroQol Plenary Meeting: Barcelona, Spain, 1995

2.8 REFERENCES

Badia X, Fernandez E, Segura A. Influence of sociodemographic and health status variables on valuation of health states in a Spanish population. European Journal of Public Health 1995;5(2):87-93.

Bergner M, Bobitt R A, Kressel S, Pollard W E, Gilson B S and Morris J R . The Sickness Impact Profile: conceptual formulation and methodology for the development of a health status measure. International Journal of Health Services 1976;6(2):393-415.

Brooks R. Health status measurement: a perspective on change. Hampshire: Macmillan Press Ltd, 1995.

van Dalen H, Williams A and Gudex C. Lay people's evaluations of health: are there variations between different subgroups? Journal of Epidemiology and Community Health 1994;48:248-253.

Gudex C. Are we lacking a dimension of energy in the EuroQol Instrument? In Bjork S (ed). EuroQol Conference Proceedings, Lund, October 1991. IHE Working Paper 92:2. Lund, Swedish Institute for Health Economics 1992:61-72.

Hunt S and McEwen J. The development of a subjective health indicator. Social Health and Illness 1980;2:231-246.

Kind P and Gudex C. Measuring health status in the community: a comparison of methods. Journal of Epidemiology and Community Health 1991;48:86-91.

Patrick D L, Bush J W and Chen M M. Methods for measuring levels of well-being for a health status index. Health Services Research 1973;8:228-245.

Patrick D L and Erickson P. Health status and health policy: quality of life in health care evaluation and resource allocation. New York: Oxford University Press, 1993.

Rosser R and Kind P. A scale of valuations of states of illness: is there a social consensus? International Journal of Epidemiology 1978;7:347-358.

Sintonen H. An approach to measuring and valuing health states. Social Science and Medicine 1981;15c:55-65.

3
The number of levels in the descriptive system

Heleen van Agt and Gouke Bonsel

3.1 INTRODUCTION

Most of us - at least the "oldies" - will remember the lengthy discussions on the current descriptive system. Many efforts have been spent on:

(i) the choice of domains,
(ii) the number of levels - if any -within a domain and
(iii) the descriptive texts themselves.

The discussion about the number of levels within a domain has a particularly long history. This research note presents a 5-level division of each domain, preceded by a short overview of arguments, which may be valid in the discussion.

3.2 OPERATIONALIZATION OF A DOMAIN

Conventional technique

Any explicitly described domain of a health status descriptive system may be operationalized in several ways. The conventional mode is to select a number of different, though related statements which together (are assumed to) cover the respective domain. Items selected this way have no natural ordering (although of course particular combinations may be strongly dependent). Usually weights are attached to each positive (however defined) response and a domain-specific score is calculated by summation of the weighted positive responses. It is essential to understand that a different weight has an interpretation according to the method which was used to retrieve weights (e.g. it could mean "relative severity as judged by laymen in a (item) pairwise comparison"). A different weight (of this type) does not mean that a positive response on the item with the highest weight implicitly or explicitly predicts response on other items of that particular domain with lower weights. In other words: conventional weighing of items has little if anything to do with empirically found ordered patterns of response.

P. Kind et al. (eds.), EQ-5D concepts and methods, 29–33.

Guttman scaling

If a descriptive system is also to be used for valuation purposes, it necessarily (in our opinion) requires another mode of domain operationalization. Just one feature of the domain is selected and items are stated in an ordered fashion, e.g. the mobility domain is represented by the feature 'walking' and the following three graded items may be formulated: 'no problems with walking', 'occasionally problems with walking', 'severe problems with walking' or 'walking no longer possible'. More levels are of course possible. This technique has some distinct advantages and disadvantages compared to the conventional approach. The conventional approach is the standard in psychological questionnaire design and follows the classical test theory. The approach described here essentially represents the development of an ordered or Guttman scale.

Advantages and disadvantages

Two major advantages of ordered scaling are: face validity, and suitability for straightforward derivation of health scenarios to be valued with an explicit valuation technique. The major disadvantages of an ordered scale are: incomplete or selected domain coverage (lack of content validity), inferior reliability, inferior precision, increased language problems, and finally higher sensitivity for the existence of impossible combinations of domain-scores if - as is usually the case in health status scales - domains are empirically dependent.

Advantages

The face validity argument is extremely important in the context of EuroQol-application. We can learn from clinical examples (APGAR, NYHA, Child-Pugh) and health measure examples (Spitzer's Q, Karnofsky, Katz's ADL, COOP-charts) that the implementation and acceptance of these non-physical measurement devices is enhanced by ordered scales. Even if an instrument gives seriously misleading numbers (Child Pugh in liver disease) it may not be replaced by superior alternatives (there are several in liver disease) because of its appealing simplicity. Perhaps the resemblance to the "real" physical scales plays a role. The suitability for derivation of health scenarios is a characteristic which bothers only the psychometricians in a health economics setting (in The Netherlands these form a small minor minority). We know that the NHP, SF-36, and SIP will never be suitable for economic valuation tasks for this reason, although it may be conceivable that some quantitative relationship exists between valuation scores of EuroQol/QWB/Rosser Kind and item-patterns of NHP/SF-36/SIP (see also Björk), where both are retrieved from the same individuals. A particular aspect of this suitability is the number of levels of the descriptive system. More levels are associated with an increasing number of possible combinations (empirical dependency excluded) which enhances the precision of the instrument as a whole (a 3^5 space consists of 243 units, a 5^5 space of 3125 units), which in turn increases the opportunities for estimation techniques to fill in validly the universe from a partial set of observations (technical quality), and which increases the opportunities for application in clinical trials. It is for these latter two reasons that the Rotterdam Group has been advocating an increase in the number of levels, if necessary at the cost of the number of domains.

Two further observations may be made:

(i) If we look at existing alternatives to EuroQol, the number of levels is higher (QWB: all domains 5; Rosser-Kind: 4+7; Rotterdam-old: 5). The descriptive COOP also has 5 levels per domain.

(ii) Not all domains require the same number of levels, but for many reasons it seems a preferable point of departure (the old EuroQol Instrument did not fulfil this requirement).

Disadvantages

The first disadvantage arises from the fact that an ordered scale, consists of one domain-specific item followed by a strictly ordered response. As we have thus far represented one domain by one item, comprehensiveness of the domain (and of the domains together) depends on the comprehensiveness of the item selected. This evidently carries a serious risk: coverage of the domain is incomplete. A natural way out is to formulate global, two- or even multi-component items as in EuroQol, but this strategy easily gives rise to the following problems: for a set of components (e.g. washing, dressing, pain, symptoms, anxious, depressed) the response may be different for the respective components. In the three-level case a solution might be: no A, no B; A or B; A and B (A and B being two aspects such as washing and dressing); but this solution in fact is a trivial and dangerous alternative to two (or more if C, D,... are added) separate dichotomous questions. The incomplete coverage may only be compensated by extension of the number of domains, a strategy which may be recognized in the early EuroQol-version (It is a matter of taste whether we call something a domain: we could also ask two instead of one domain-specific question). The second disadvantage is lack of reliability. Reliability of 2 5-level questions is (by definition almost) lower than that of 5 dichotomous questions, although the number of response-units (10) is the same. The precision, related to the theoretical number of different responses, is much greater in the multi-item case: in the above-mentioned example 25 states versus 1024 states. Finally, again by definition, the risk of restrictive interactions is highest in ordered scales, particularly if the number of domains is high. (E.g. observable in EuroQol, early version)

3.3 HOW TO INCREASE THE NUMBER OF LEVELS

Grading may be achieved by choosing a suitable principle, by stating the ceiling/floor sensitivity and by finding the right nomenclature.

Grading principles

Grading in the health status context may be according to "severity", "disturbance", "need for assistance" (not always applicable), "frequency", and so forth. We would suggest adherence to the "severity" principle.

Ceiling/floor sensitivity

Given a stated number of levels ($n \geq 3$), an important choice concerns the refinement of measurement on the full axis from extremely unhealthy to healthy. The refinement can be different for different parts of the axis. If, e.g., 3 out of 4 levels cover infrequent, rather unhealthy states, the ceiling sensitivity is low, and, as a consequence, the probability of detecting change is, in most practical low-morbidity circumstances, also low. This characteristic is of course influenced by the test-population(s) for which the instrument will be used, but particularly if generic use is aimed at, ceiling sensitivity should be sufficient. Note that 'equidistant' stratification is a rather nonsensical term without an external (quantitative) criterion to judge equidistance - which in our case may be derived from modeling exercises like those of Ben van Hout presented in Lund. Here we present two versions, the first being a five-level normal version and the other being a five-level ceiling-sensitive version.

The right nomenclature

In The Netherlands extensive research has been devoted to the meaning of words such as 'moderate'. Many words with a natural ordering - according to the well-educated psychometrician - and a natural context of use, appeared to have other meanings and connotations in random samples of the general population by contrast with the psychological student population. In our case the same problem applies, to which the problem of translation should also be added. The versions presented here should be judged carefully in this regard.

3.4 TWO VERSIONS

In Table 3.1 there are two versions of EuroQol distinguishing 5 levels in each domain.

Table 3.1 5-dimensional EuroQol questionaire

Cat.	Categories 1-4 equidistant	Categories 1-5 equidistant
	Walking about	
1	no problems in	no problems in
2	practically no problems in / very small problems in / very little problems in	practically no problems in / very small problems in / very little problems in
3	small / slight / minor / somewhat problems in	some problems in / rather problems in
4	some problems in / rather problems in	many problems in / only able in...with crutch or walking frame
5	unable to walk about / confined to bed or wheelchair	rumble to walk about / confined to bed or wheelchair
	Washing or dressing self	
1	no problems with	no problems with
2	practically no problems with / very small problems with / very little problems with	practically no problems with / very small problems with / very little problems with
3	small / slight / minor / somewhat problems with	some problems in / rather problems with
4	some problems with / rather problems with	many problems with
5	tumble to wash or dress self	unable to wash or drew self
	Usual activities (e.g. work, study, housework. family or Leisure activities)	
1	no problems with	no problems with
2	practically no problems with / very small problems with / very little problems with	practically no problems with / very small problems with / very little problems with
3	small / slight / minor / somewhat problems with	some problems in / rather problems with
4	some problems with / rather problems with	many problems with
5	unable to perform	unable to perform
	Pain or discomfort	
1	no	no
2	practically no / occasionally light	practically no / occasionally light
3	mild	moderate
4	moderate	severe
5	extreme	extreme
	Anxious or depressed	
1	not	not
2	little	little
3	slightly I somewhat	moderately
4	moderately	very
5	extremely	extremely

Presented at the EuroQol Plenary Meeting: Rotterdam, The Netherlands, 1993

4

First steps to assessing semantic equivalence of the EuroQol Instrument: Results of a questionnaire survey to members of the EuroQol Group

Julia Fox-Rushby

4.1 INTRODUCTION

Increasing worldwide interest in using outcome measures to inform decision-making in the health sector has encouraged the translation of HRQoL instruments from the language in which they were developed (usually some form of English) to other languages. One of the early effects of this was that the developers of instruments found several versions of their instrument in another language. Following this, developers of HRQoL instruments have been relatively quick to provide guidance on how to standardise the translation process, and also to encourage translators to maintain links with themselves. At present the groups who developed the following generic instruments (Sickness Impact Profile (SIP), Short Form 36 (SF-36), WHOQOL, Nottingham Health Profile (NHP)) have all created 'guidelines' for translation. Alongside these developments there have been a number of papers categorising notions of 'equivalence' that 'should' be attained (see for example: Bullinger *et al*, 1993; Touw-Otten and Meadows, 1996; Sartorius and Kuyken, 1994) as well as debating how to decrease the costs of the process (Mathias *et al*, 1994). Attention is now turning to questioning the principles on which the 'guidance' is based and towards examining procedures used for translation within other disciplines (Fox-Rushby and Parker, 1995; Herdman *et al*, 1997).

A paper presented for discussion at the EuroQol conference in 1995 (Fox-Rushby and Badia, 1996) described, and reflected upon, the development of international language versions of the EuroQol Instrument. This paper concluded that a principal 'challenge' to the Group was "to directly assess conceptual equivalence between the English language version and each of the other language versions". The Group is currently in the position (once again) of being asked to 'endorse' the translation of the EuroQol Instrument for use in at least five further countries (including Japan, Russia and Italy). It would appear, then, that the need to contemplate the process of translation and meaning of the EuroQol Instrument in other languages will not disappear - indeed it is being encouraged in the EuroQol Manual. As part of the recommendations for examining the degree of 'equivalence' it was suggested (Fox-Rushby and Badia, 1996) that "providing definitions of key terms in the EuroQol Instrument" could be a way forward. Whilst this paper focuses on the EuroQol Instrument, many

P. Kind et al. (eds.), EQ-5D concepts and methods, 35–52.

of the problems and issues raised will have resonance for the developers and users of other generic measures of HRQoL.

The suggestion to seek ways of rewriting the EuroQol Instrument is not new within the translation field. However, it is based on a key assumption; that we would like the meaning of the EuroQol Instrument to be understood in different languages i.e. that we are seeking to promote a meaning based translation, rather than a literal translation. As Barnwell (1992) states, this may;
"1) change the order of the words; it will use the order which is most clear and natural in the language into which the translation is being made; 2) change the expressions or the idioms; it will use the words which give the same meaning as the original clearly, even though this may not be the same idiom as in the original message".

One effect of this assumption is that translation itself, as Larson (1984) suggested, begins with the source text (in this case the EuroQol Instrument itself) and analysing this text into a semantic structure. It is suggested that the translator begins to identify key words or phrases so that "the components of meaning which are crucial and need to be transferred (are) identified". This involves both searching for lexical equivalents as well as semantic rewrites of text. The principal advantage of this process is that "most of the implicit information is made explicit and the secondary and figurative senses eliminated". Therefore, this enhances the probability of an 'accurate' transfer of meaning.

Given that notions of 'health' are varied and complex; that the EuroQol members helping translators have often been unsure of how to choose from a range of words in other languages; that the people responsible for categorising and describing health in the EuroQol Instrument are the development group themselves, rather than members of the public; and because I assumed the EuroQol Group would prefer to establish meaning themselves rather than have translators in different countries assume it, a questionnaire was sent round to existing members of the EuroQol Group who were involved in the development of the EuroQol Instrument . This chapter reports the results of the questionnaire survey on the meaning of key words in the EuroQol Instrument, by members of the EuroQol Group. Responses revealed a range of alternative words/phrases as well as a range of implicit meanings/assumptions. It also showed that contradictory views were held within the Group. The paper recommends that the EuroQol Group clarifies the questions raised and takes some decisions regarding translation of the EuroQol Instrument in the future.

4.2 METHODS

A questionnaire was sent out in January 1996 to existing members of the EuroQol Group who had been involved during various stages of the development of the EuroQol Instrument (n=23). The aim of the questionnaire was to elicit a clearer understanding of key terms and phrases within the original English language version of the EuroQol Instrument[1] in order to facilitate the process of translation and improve the possibility of creating semantically equivalent questionnaires in other languages.

The 'key terms/phrases' were chosen on the basis of whether: terms had proved difficult to translate (such as self-care, extreme); terms used to categorise people's health state (both in titles and descriptors e.g. mobility / walking about); and the centrality of an idea to understanding valuation (such as best/worst imaginable health state). Each person was asked to write about what they thought the EuroQol Group meant to convey by a set of words or phrases. Telephone reminders were made in January and reminder letters were faxed to the remaining people in July, and again in September.

Responses were tabulated by term/phrase and each item was considered in relation to: the most common idea presented; whether there were specific items included or excluded; the range of alternative words proposed; whether any contrasting ideas were presented; whether there were any other important notions portrayed within the responses; the level of specificity of answers; number of missing responses, or responses using the same word as the original text; and any immediately obvious implications for translation.

4.3 RESULTS

Of the 23 questionnaires sent out, 20 were returned by the 23rd September 1996. Of these, 3 returned only the first page and one form was 'spoilt'. The response rate for each question was high, with the exceptions of best and 'worst imaginable health state' and the last long phrase concerning health after 1 year. Few alternative phrases/words were elicited for the state dead, walking about and best/worst imaginable health state. Finally, a common response contained questions either about what should be included or what the Group had originally intended for inclusion. The summaries for each of the words/phrases are shown below and are followed by a summary of spontaneous comments received.

'Health' / 'Your own health state'

Quite a range of categorisations was given. Most respondents wrote something along the lines of physical, psychological and social well-being. Those that did not stated "health care related health", "enjoyment of life despite presence of health condition" and "absence of illness". Two notable exclusions were made: "wider connotations of health" and "social well-being". There were a number of contrasting ideas presented including: those that concentrated on the words 'well-being' versus 'functioning'; those who specifically mentioned the WHO definition versus those who only defined

1. Which was the base language version used for all EuroQol Group discussions

'health' in terms of the EuroQol dimensions; one wrote that health was the absence of illness, whereas another stated that, even with illness, health was whether a person can enjoy life; another felt that health should not be a medical term, whereas another said it should be health care related health. Not surprisingly, with such broad notions, people did not furnish their answers with elaborate specification.

The responses to the phrase 'your own health state' mostly referred to 'health' but emphasis was on a person's own judgement of themselves. It was based on autonomy and individuality, and the sense that one's own health depended on one's own situation. People stated that it could either be broader or narrower than the EuroQol Group's view of 'health'.

'Today'

This was mostly described as referring to the day of completing the questionnaire (e.g. this day, this particular calendar day, current 24 hours). However, people also noted that it could either be shorter than 24 hours and mean "this moment", "waking hours" or longer "presently: more or less representative of a short period (last week)".

'A person like you'

Four people said it would be the person completing the questionnaire. One person wrote "someone with my personal characteristics in my personal situation", which I also interpret as 'myself'. The other type of responses incorporated two sets of ideas; firstly that it was someone with the same socio-demographic characteristics (such as age, sex, and possibly the following - education, employment, region, social status, and health state); secondly, that it was someone who had the same "value system", which seems to be alternatively described as "obligations and interests", "holding the same moral, philosophical and spiritual values", and "of similar temperament when thinking more generally".

Some opposite views drawn from the responses included: first, whether it is a question of socio- demographics only or not; second whether it included the same health state (or health history) or not. It is interesting that one respondent split up a value system according to whether thinking about health or 'more generally'. Finally, it is noteworthy that some socio-demographic variables listed in defining 'person like you' are not included in the last page of the EuroQol Instrument long form questionnaire.

'Personal view'

Other words used for personal were: 'a person like you', subjective, one, respondent, own, self, and I. Alternatives for view were opinion, think, thoughts, and perception. The only exclusion stated was that this would not include "partner, parents, or Her

Majesty the Queen". The only other idea presented was that such a statement implied there were no right or wrong answers.

'Self-Care'

The most common idea presented was that self-care was about washing and dressing (six responses just had this). Seventeen responses mentioned at least washing and dressing. Other actions included were feeding, going to the toilet, grooming, brushing teeth and also providing oneself with drinks and food. Some specific activities noted for exclusion were social and role activities, and one person questioned whether continence and transfer should be included in this category. There was considerable agreement about this category, although nine people provided examples not currently covered by the English version of the EuroQol Instrument.

The important underlying idea of this dimension seems to point towards independence in basic daily care activities. The level of specificity was fairly general, although three people gave quite detailed examples, such as "hand or foot care", "brushing teeth", and "can wipe own bottom".

'Mobility'

The main idea presented encompassed the ability to move from one place to another, and not just by walking. Other forms allowing movement were by wheelchair, driving and 'transport'. Contrasting opinions expressed were whether the Group actually meant just walking/being ambulant or not. Other ideas used to clarify this debate centre on the effect i.e. "to accomplish tasks freely without hindrance" or "capacity to move" rather than actual movement.

There was little detail. Most answers concentrated on moving, without giving any details of how. The few that did were either contradictory, or gave additional alternatives to walking. Finally, one person did highlight an inconsistency between the word used for the dimension and the words used in statements. The word used to describe the dimension (mobility) implies a general term for movement, whereas the levels concentrate on ability to walk.

'Walking about'

The most common idea presented involved walking about on two feet. Other ideas included why people would walk and how they would know if they could walk without problems. These centred around being able to walk for daily activities and also being able to walk without constraints (e.g. having to stop, using a wheelchair, and 'difficulties'). However, walking about for one person included "any steps taken even with crutches, walking frames or support". There were some definite exclusions given, such as 'strenuous activities', 'country walks', and 'sport' and one answer also excluded arm movements.

Independence in walking appeared to be a highly valued state by the EuroQol Group, as well as being able to walk where someone wants to walk without physical or psychological hindrance. Some responses raised the question of where people moving around in wheelchairs should be located on the EuroQol Instrument, with suggestions that they would be excluded from walking without any/some difficulty (although debate during the EuroQol conference questioned whether this was appropriate).

'Confined to bed'

The main idea conveyed was of being restricted to bed and only able to move out of bed with some help. However, the actual range of answers lay between "unable to get out of bed without help" and "not able to go outdoors, even with help". The majority of queries were raised about the extent of mobility and whether a person would be able to get to a toilet by themselves or not. The range of answers covered "use of a bedpan", "can, but only with considerable help", "possibly able to use toilet" and one response suggested it depended on how people relate it to the previous question about walking. The notion of dependency is crucial to the question but it would appear that the actual level is viewed differently and may need to be clarified and agreed by the Group prior to further translation.

Other ideas were included in the answers. For example, one person felt that a chair could be thought of instead of just a bed. Three people mentioned causes for staying in bed: "as a result of any medical condition, because of some health problem or just required to stay in bed". This latter person was particularly interesting because there was a further qualification: "not just lying there because tired, not literally tied to the bed". Two answers included some further commentary about time: one stating "more or less for the entire day" and another "on the day of the interview". Finally, no one used the English word 'confined'.

This phrase has created some problems in translation but, as long as the EuroQol Group can agree the level or range of specificity, it should be possible ensure that the category is subject to a smaller range of interpretations.

'Usual Activities'

The predominant sense conveyed by the responses was that this centred on daily activities such as work, study, leisure, and social activities (all written as examples in the original English version) of the EuroQol Instrument. The statements given were mostly inclusive rather than exclusive and it appears to be a very broad category. The only exclusion given was "activities other than self-care". Contrasting ideas presented occurred in two themes; firstly whether 'usual' meant 'daily' or 'regular', and secondly whether it included 'role' or other activities. This was most clearly exemplified by one respondent who wrote "habitual or regular activities; not necessarily 'normal' because others may not do them; not necessarily 'daily' but just regular e.g. Bingo on Thursdays".

Other ideas presented were that it referred to activities preceding illness, and whether a person felt fulfilled or not. There was little specificity in responses, with the exception of one respondent. One area for clarification is the notion of how regular is 'usual'. Whilst the majority of answers pointed to daily, there are clearly important questions for translation if usual can mean less than daily.

'Pain'

Fourteen people used the word pain to describe pain! However, other words also given included hurt, aches, personal suffering, acute discomfort, intense somatic discomfort and, more unusually, breathlessness. Despite this, some people specifically excluded these words e.g. pain is "stronger than ache". There were few other ideas presented. One mentioned intensity; pain "ranges from short/sharp to deep and chronic". Others centred on its effect both on self-care/mobility and usual activities as well as whether pain requires relief or not. There was very little specificity in response to this word.

'Discomfort'

Generally, it appeared that people struggled to describe discomfort: that they weren't quite sure what the EuroQol Group meant. There was quite a wide range of replies, which seem to fall into two main categories; those who said discomfort was intense pain and those who included non-pain physical sensations. Not surprisingly therefore, a number of contradictions were highlighted. These included whether discomfort only concerned physical or also psychological and/or physical disturbances; whether discomfort was something which could be 'disregarded' or not; and whether physical comfort was about how you felt about physical discomfort.

Some of the ideas presented covered whether people were able to adapt to discomfort or not and that discomfort was something not as intense or acute as pain. The overall responses tended to be non-specific. When people did give examples, the most frequently cited was itching, followed by pain, aches, nausea and tiredness. Others mentioned were dizziness, bloatedness, pins and needles, and ringing in ears.

'Anxiety/anxious'

The principal idea used was one of 'worry'. Other words used were; dread, distress, tenseness, troubled, fear/afraid, panic, nervous, and apprehension. One person did, however, state that anxiety was stronger/deeper/longer than nervous/worry. Other ideas mainly raised issues of cause and effect. People stated that this category could include anxiety from a number of causes ("both non-clinical worries and clinical anxiety", "worry about paying a telephone bill to fear/panic attacks", "general state - anxious person- or specific e.g. diagnosis, uncertainty of future or phobia/panic"). The effects of anxiety were described as disturbing normal living, causing particular physical symptoms, and affecting one's ability to enjoy life. Any specificity in the responses tended to concentrate on possible causes.

'Depressed'

The principal notion written about concerned being unhappy/low. Other words chosen were; blue, miserable, cheerless, gloomy, dejected, withdrawn, down, sad, hopeless, and misery. Contrasting opinions concerned whether this was about clinical depression or not, or whether it included both. Other ideas raised issues of time, cause, and effect. Time was used as a way of defining whether a person was depressed or not, and principally that depression "was not .... just a day or two" and that it was "in excess of a week". As with anxiety, cause was attributed to a whole variety of factors from "having an argument with someone which leaves the subject feeling 'low' to clinically diagnosed depression" and "with or without reason". Effects were described as "interferes with social relationships, subject unable to enjoy life in any area" and "unable to do things normally would do".

Two people did not complete this question and two used the same word. The level of specificity was limited to broad feelings, with few specific examples, and thus little further illumination. However, this was one example where several alternative words were given to the actual word itself.

'Some problems'

Quite a wide range of descriptions and ideas were given in response to these words. The main notion was that it implied a range from a small number/degree of difficulty to severe difficulties. It was primarily given a meaning concerning frequency of problems, with people giving examples such as "not daily", "chronic number 1-3" "small number", "more than 1 problem", "every now and then", and "from 1 to many". Some respondents felt that it was not an indication of severity. Other ways that people tried to explain 'some problems' was in terms of how people would react ("problems which may need medical intervention, independent problems which do not compromise subject's ability to self-care"; "they would be noticeable to the individual"; "unable to perform task/activity as would wish"; "problems do not overcrowd normal life, bearable").

'Moderate'

The responses to this were similar to 'some problems', but people seemed to have given more specific 'locations' to the 'degree'. One respondent, for example, wrote 30%. There were, however some contrasting views, and these specifically relate to the 'positioning' of the word. For example, "towards lower end of pain scale" vs. "middling to bad" vs. "central tendency" vs. "somewhat above average".

One respondent also raised problems concerning translation. 'Moderate' is clearly an inexact idea. If something was back translated as 'in between none and very much', how would the EuroQol Group feel? If it were not acceptable the concept needs to be defined more carefully in English or possibly a different word chosen.

'Extreme'

'Very severe' was the most commonly used rewording, although other words used were 'very much', 'very very strong', 'a lot', and 'very high degree of'. Other indications were given to exemplify, and included 'almost intolerable', 'life almost not worth living', '100% of the problem'. There were a range of different, and contrasting ideas presented (e.g. could be strong feelings or bad problems; most a person and/or others could imagine, that it is a 'range rather than a point).

'Best/worst imaginable health state'

The main ideas presented for 'best imaginable health state' were optimal/ideal health state a person can think of. Other words used for best were: very good, best level, well, and most. Phrases used for 'worst' were: very bad; alive but that's all; unable to function independently in all areas of life; as bad as it is possible to be; presence of all dysfunction in human system compatible with life; serious limiting consequences.

In describing the 'best', some resorted to their previous definitions of health, thus similar ideas are repeated here: absence of dysfunction; capacity of perform; fully occupied living. Contrasting beliefs highlighted were whether or not the health state imagined was influenced by the EuroQol Instrument itself. Other issues raised were that the respondent may or may not have experienced their best imaginable state, whilst one person questioned whether it existed or not. This leads to the more worrying aspect of the responses; there were three missing responses and two 'don't knows', with one person going as far as saying "never really had much idea and don't know". In addition to this many people used the same words (best, worst, health state, or imaginable) somewhere in their description. One response gave notably vivid examples for 'worst imaginable health state': "meningococcus septic shock, big bullae, losing your skin, extreme pain, knowing you will die in 4-5 hours ..... the horror of a six year old crushed by a potato van on the lower half of the body, dying and half conscious".

'Unconscious'

The predominant idea conveyed by respondents was that unconscious meant being alive but not awake, and not aware of surroundings. The responses were interesting in that a range of ways of describing this were given, although one person wrote that they had to recourse to a dictionary! Beyond the ideas summarised, people described how one could tell if someone was unconscious; not reacting to pain, eyes closed, breathing spontaneously, cannot actively think, and dependent on others for life support. Only one person gave an exclusion; "it does not include delirium or confusion". Other ideas raised focused principally on time and included; "could be seconds/ months/years", "for a long time", "can be temporary or long lasting", "very short or very long time". Given that the EuroQol Instrument stipulates 1 year, it was quite surprising that particularly those who chose to mention time did not mention this. People tended to give fairly specific answers to this question.

'The state dead'

Not surprisingly the most common idea was of being no longer alive! However, it is interesting that two very specific exclusions were given; that it did not include the process of dying; and that there is no assumption of an after life. In relation to the latter point there were some contrasting views of death - that the Group assumes just release from a physical life or "state of no return" versus "going to the maker". Any details given to this phrase tended to concentrate on definitions of brain/heart death.

'When thinking about each health state imagine that it will last for 1 year. What happens after that is not known and is not taken into account'

There were eight responses either completely missing or the respondent said they were unable to rewrite it. The main ideas written about by the remaining twelve people was that the respondent should think about a description given for 1 year, that anything could happen after that (getting better, worse, same, die) but it is uncertain and should not be thought about. Only consider the 1 year, during which you remain in the same state. The principal idea that people tried to express was the desire to eliminate prognosis from people's thinking, although one person also commented that the discount rate after 1 year was infinity.

Spontaneous comments

Comments generally came from people in two ways; with a covering letter or written directly on to the questionnaire. There were four kinds of comments. One type covered the difficulty encountered in completing the questionnaire; one person wrote, "it was harder than expected"; another "some concepts have no equivalent, cannot be easily described or are self-evident"; other people also noted that it took longer than 20 minutes.

A second set of comments focused specifically on the definitions of anxiety/depression: one person wrote "anxiety and depression have text book definitions but I think that in these cases we feel that if patients consider themselves depressed (on their own criteria) then that is what matters"; another wrote "anxiety/depression (by concepts not clinical definition/mood concepts)".

The third group of comments made more general observations. It is interesting that two people wrote that, whilst they were trying to think what the Group meant, they also felt they had been influenced by the comments of patients completing the EuroQol Instrument. Others commented generally on meaning, for example "I think that the EuroQol Instrument aims to be comprehensive at a cost of specificity so, once again, I find that a lot of these terms can cover a wide range" and "I suppose this has confirmed what I had already guessed, namely that we are on shaky ground arguing for the 'purity' of the English language version. However, I think that you can take the 'gestalt' view of the content, in which case the detail of the language itself becomes less of a problem".

4.4 DISCUSSION

One of the principal findings of the questionnaire was that it highlights a whole range of implicit meanings that will be helpful for translating the EuroQol Instrument into other languages in the future. For example, anxiety/anxious does not only refer to a clinically defined state, mobility does refer to walking as well as other movement, and the state dead does not refer to the process of dying. Such ideas have been gathered by focusing not only on what is included, but on what is excluded. It is also likely that an external professional translator would not have derived this range of implicit meanings, since they would not have had access to the discussions of past years. Whilst many of the 'implicit' meanings may not be a surprise to members of the EuroQol Group, they are not ideas that are readily accessible by researchers outside the Group. The exposure of implicit understandings can only help to facilitate understanding of what the EuroQol Instrument is trying to measure and as different types of information are held explicit or implicit in different languages, a semantic re-write may improve decisions made in other languages.

Secondly, it is clear that there are particular words/phrases that the Group is in close agreement with such as 'today' and, surprisingly given the difficulties encountered in translation, 'self-care'. This would suggest that we should not be so concerned with the latter as there seems to be a fairly good impression that it is about washing and dressing all parts of the body by oneself, possibly also being able to feed oneself (although not necessarily able to prepare the food). It would also suggest that translating the words 'self-care' need not be adhered to so closely as there is a good understanding of what the concept covers. With regard to 'today', again there seems to be a widely held view that this relates to 24 hours surrounding the completion of the questionnaire. Given this, the Dutch version should be questioned as it uses a different time period (back translated as last week) and consider whether it should be changed if there is a suitable Dutch word. Thirdly, several alternative words/phrases have been suggested, which should help the process of choosing words in alternative languages.

The 'success' of the exercise could be questioned on two grounds, although future action could alleviate the majority of concerns. First some words/phrases were given very few alternatives e.g. pain. In such cases future translators have effectively been given little to work with, although the situation could be improved through recourse to lexicons and dictionaries. However this situation itself could cause us to ponder on our own understanding of the EuroQol Instrument and as a Group we could be challenged by the idea that others may find it even more difficult to explain, or understand. Such questions have prompted me to wonder why people did not offer alternatives and I suggest there may be a range of reasons: first, a self-completed questionnaire is not an ideal research method for an examination of meaning and personal interviews or small discussion groups are more likely to elicit both more and better quality information; second, there could be a reluctance to question the existing EuroQol Instrument or a belief that the English language is so exact and precise in meaning that to change some words/phrases would alter the whole meaning and render incomparable alternative English versions of the EuroQol Instrument (rather like a controlled scientific experiment); third, a belief that the group has one mind on the issue or that the people completing the EuroQol Instrument are of like mind to the EuroQol developers; or finally, that having been part of the Group for so long it is actually too difficult to think outside of the frame of the EuroQol Instrument and that the EuroQol Group has become isolated from explanation and has no point of comparison to aid description.

Secondly, the 'success' could be questioned on the basis that there are contradictory views demonstrated between Group members (e.g. for discomfort), as well as there being direct questions raised about what is (or not) included (e.g. mobility). In one sense this is surprising, as the Group has worked together on the instrument since 1986. However, there are several other reasons it could be expected; first the view of a group is likely to change over time; secondly, the context (asking individuals to think of the group view) is likely to produce variety; thirdly, Group members will hold different views individually which reflect personal experiences of life, and an instrument developed by a group will represent a compromise of opinions; fourthly, some people said they had been influenced by the interpretation of people completing the EuroQol Instrument whilst others may have been influenced by more regular use of alternative language versions; and finally, studies of meaning will always uncover the ambiguities of language. The reasons for why views differ would be fascinating in themselves. However, these findings do allow us to discuss and agree the range of attributable meanings desired (or not) as a Group, based on our understanding at present. It also shows the potential impact that any one person could have on the versions of the EuroQol Instrument produced in other languages and the importance of documenting fuller descriptions at the development stage of instruments.

Whilst this chapter has focused on meaning, to aid translation, it can also be used to raise questions about the choice of English in the original language version. An early assumption of this work was that we were aiming for a 'meaning' based translation and not a literal translation (where word for word translations are used as far as possible). As Newmark (1988) states, one of the consequences of this is that the translated text may well read better than the original text and certainly better than a literal translation. This leads me to question just how 'bound' we should feel to the original English version, as one of the spontaneous comments received intimated. If the EuroQol Group is concerned with 'meaning' and other languages can move away from literal translations, what implications does this have for the original English text?

In the future, I suggest the EuroQol Group takes decisions and action in the following areas: first, on specific issues of semantics; the additional use of dictionaries and lexicons to extend the range of alternative words and phrases; for the EuroQol Group to agree the meaning of selected terms and phrases on the basis of categories which raise important contradictions, where people asked direct questions as well as those which have caused particular difficulty in translation to date; secondly, to ascertain the extent to which the general public view the meanings of key words/phrases, and how this varies across space and time; thirdly, to consider general issues concerning the translation of the EuroQol Instrument. For example, to decide on the level of importance the Group wishes, and is able to give, to the issue of translation; and to agree a translation protocol, which is clearly linked to particular notions of 'equivalence'. Finally, to decide whether the EuroQol Group is interested in pursuing the use of the EuroQol Instrument as a tool to investigate issues of translation of HRQL instruments *per se* (as it does issues of valuation).

Finally, I leave you with the thoughts of one of the respondents ...

"I'm not sure if (you have) opened Pandora's box or a can of worms, but it can only be a most illuminating and productive exercise."

4.5 POSTSCRIPT

I wrote this paper four years ago for two main reasons: first, to help ease some of the problems in translating the EuroQol Instrument; and secondly to help question the thinking involved in the international translation of HRQoL instruments generally - both in the 'how' and the 'why'. It was influenced by my experiences in considering the relevance of existing generic HRQoL measures to the Mukamba and Maragoli of Kenya, and our attempts to develop a measure of HRQoL based on local conceptions of health (Fox-Rushby *et al*, 1995 and 1997). Our early research showed that not only was it difficult to translate health-related terms into the two languages but also that - even when translation was done carefully and sensitively - terms took on meanings that related to culturally specific premises and to their use in specific contexts (Amuyunzu *et al*, 1995; Allen *et al*, 1997).

The translation work in the HRQoL field (not just within the EuroQol Group) did not appear to recognise these issues. Part of the reason why I believe this to be the case is because both the users and developers of the majority of generic HRQoL instruments treat these tools (either explicitly or implicitly) as if they were 'culture-free' when in fact they are 'culture-full', reflecting in particular the beliefs and values of the researchers who developed them (Fox-Rushby and Parker, 1995). Therefore it is important to understand that the translation of HRQoL instruments is not instrumental only in the transportation of words, but also of the ideas and culture embodied within the source language (and hence the culture of the original researchers).

Such thinking is the starting point for Robinson's critique of translation studies, where he weaves inextricable links between translation and colonial domination (Robinson, 1997). From such a position, the translation of HRQoL questionnaires represents a form of neo-colonialism. Such views may be considered 'extreme' in the HRQoL field, where the majority of researchers work from a premise of 'universal' conceptions of 'health' (Fox-Rushby and Parker, 1995). Grounds for criticism of such views are well documented by the renowned Kenyan writer Ngugi Wa Thiong'o. In a series of essays he (Wa Thiong'o, 1993a) argues that what tends to be represented as 'universal' is in fact 'eurocentric' and that eurocentricsm is therefore anti-universalist. As he states "I am suspicious of the uses of the word and the concept universal. For very often, this has meant the West generalising its experience in history as the universal experience of the world. What is Western becomes universal and what is Third World becomes local" (Wa Thiong'o, 1993b). However, his thinking is still that of a universalist in that he believes there is a 'centre' to world thinking, but that it is not represented in the ideas currently conveyed.

Given such texts and our dissatisfaction with both translation guidelines as well as the practice of translation in the HRQoL field, collaboration within the EuroQol Group led to two papers (Herdman *et al*, 1997 and 1998). The first outlined alternative philosophical positions regarding universalism, absolutism and relativism and the links with approaches taken to translation. It also showed the considerable confusion of terminology in the field. The second paper developed a model of 'equivalence' from the viewpoint of universalism, and suggested a range of methods for investigating each type of 'equivalence'.

This paper was therefore written to facilitate the investigation of equivalence, and the extent to which notions of health represented in existing HRQoL measures are universal. I recognise that it is a very small step, and that criticisms would be justified from the alternative schools of thought in translation studies, and different disciplinary branches in linguistics. For example, given Fawcett (1997) I am concerned that slicing words out of the EuroQol Instrument may not help translation if other languages choose to slice up sentences in different ways. It may encourage translation to focus too much on words or phrases rather than sentences and then beyond to the overall context. Depending on the way 'meaning' is described, it may also lead people into believing only one meaning exists, when in fact meaning may be open to many interpretations. Equally, the methods cannot be said to be capable of providing sensitive insights into each EuroQol members' views and there was evidence of some unwillingness to participate. It remains to be seen whether such pragmatic approaches can be used to increase consensus about meanings on an international basis.

Since this paper was written there have been many changes with respect to translation of the EuroQol Instrument (I do not claim this to be a causal link). There are now many more translated versions available, particularly for pages 2-3. A translation protocol has been written and modified over time (most recently to allow more questioning of what respondents think about when answering the questions), and a list of intended meanings for key words and phrases on pages 2-3 was put forward to the EuroQol Group this year - although there was not time in the meeting to reach any agreement. Translations have also been undertaken from the Spanish Castillian version, rather than the English questionnaire, for use in Latin America. Finally translation was one of the three main areas of the European Union Biomed grant held by the EuroQol Group.

Any questioning of meaning can be challenging, and suggestions of change to an established instrument met with resistance. The role of translation in this process was recognised by Guyatt (1995) as he highlighted requests not to 'improve on the original-language questionnaire' during the translation (despite there being recognised deficiencies in that questionnaire). However, he also suggested developing new questions for new countries and using meta analytic methods to compare results across different countries. The EuroQol has recognised the former. To enable comparable research to continue it was agreed that no changes would be made to the EuroQol Instrument until the end of the Biomed grant in 2001, when changes will be considered in the light of results from research over the previous 11 years.

Whether the reader thinks the EuroQol Group (and more generally the developers of generic measures of HRQoL) have responded sufficiently to issues raised through translation will depend on their assumptions of what translation involves. I also recognise that any conclusions in practice will be made given the resources available. However, it would appear that the considerable resources spent on providing 'values' and population norms for different instruments points to either 'absolutism' or bad science dressed up as pragmatism claiming penury.

To allow greater understanding of the range and ambiguity of meaning, I would suggest that a carefully designed international study of respondents' understanding of the EuroQol Instrument might begin to represent and *explain* the range of meanings given. This would then allow us to understand and question the interpretations given to the increasing number of international comparisons of health states and values attributed to health states. It would also allow us to see how closely these understandings match those of the developers of instruments.

4.6 ACKNOWLEDGEMENTS

Thanks to everyone in the EuroQol Group for taking time out of their busy schedules to complete the questionnaire and to engage with some difficult issues. I am grateful to Caroline Selai, Rosalind Rabin, Frank de Charro, Xavier Badia and Michel Herdman for comments on the draft questionnaire; to Jane Pelerin for collating all the questionnaires into tables; to Glaxo for funding my travel to attend the EuroQol Meeting in Oslo; and to Ray FitzPatrick and Annabel Bowden for their comments on this chapter. Finally I acknowledge the funding of a post-doctoral fellowship from the Economic and Social Research Council (Grant No 52425094) in the UK.

Originally presented at the EuroQol Plenary Meeting: Oslo, Norway, 1996

4.7 REFERENCES

Allen T, Parker M, Amuyunzu M, Johnson K, Mwanzo I, Mwenesi H, Fox-Rushby J. Conceptions of health in quality of life research. Quality of Life Research 1997;6(7/8):614.

Amuyunzu M, Allen T, Mwenesi H, Johnson K, Egesah O, Parker M, Fox-Rushby J. The resonance of language: Health terms in Kenya. Quality of Life Research 1995;4(5):388.

Badia X, Fox-Rushby J, Herdman M. The cross-cultural adaptation and harmonisation of existing versions of the EuroQol questionnaire. A research proposal, Mimeo, 1996.

Barnwell K. Bible Translation: An introductory course in translation principles, 3rd edition, Dallas: Summer Institute of Linguistics, 1992.

Bullinger M, Anderson R, Cella D, Aaronson N. Developing and evaluating cross-cultural instruments: From minimum requirements to optimal models. Quality of Life Research 1993;2(45):1-459.

Fawcett P. Translation and language. Manchester: St Jerome Publishing, 1997.

Fox-Rushby J, Mwenesi H, Parker M, Amuyunzu M, Egesah O, Johnson K, Allen T. Questioning premises: Health-related quality of life in Kenya. Quality of Life Research 1995;5(4):428-429.

Fox-Rushby J, Badia X. Development of the international versions of the EuroQol Instrument: Challenges for the future. In: Badia X, Herdman M, Segura A, editors. EuroQol Plenary Meeting Discussion Papers 1996:123-134.

Fox-Rushby J, Johnson K, Mwanzo I, Amuyunzu M, Mwenesi H, Allen T, Parker M, Muthami M, Bowden A, Munguti K, Chiama O. Creating an instrument to assess lay perceptions of HRQL: Options and implications. Quality of Life Research 1997;6(7/8): 633.

Fox-Rushby J, Parker M. Culture and the measurement of health-related quality of life. European Review of Applied Psychology 1995;45(4):257-263.

Guyatt G H. The philosophy of translation. In: Shumaker S and Berzon R, editors. The International assessment of health-related quality of life: Theory, translation, measurement and analysis. Oxford: Rapid Communications, 1995.

Herdman M, Fox-Rushby J, Badia X. Equivalence and the translation and adaptation of health-related quality of life measures. Quality of Life Research 1997;6:237-247

Herdman M, Fox-Rushby J, Badia X. A model of equivalence in the cultural adaptation of HRQL instruments: The universalist approach. Quality of Life Research 1998;7:323-355.

Larson M L. Meaning based translation: A guide to cross-language equivalence. University Press of America, 1984.

Mathias S D, Fifer S K, Patrick D L. Rapid translation of quality of life measures for international trials: Avoiding errors of the minimalist approach. Quality of Life Research 1994;3:403-412.

Newmark P. A textbook of translation. Prentice Hall, International language teaching, 1988.

Robinson D. Translation and empire. Manchester: St Jerome Publishing, 1997.

Sartorius N, Kuyken W. Translation of health status instruments. In: Orley J, and Kuyken W, editors. Quality of life assessment: International perspectives. Heidleberg: Springer-Verlag, 1994

Touw-Otten F, Meadows K. Cross-cultural issues. In: outcome measurement. In: Hutchinson A, McColl E, Christic M, Rittleton C, editors. Outcome measurement in primary and out-patient care. Harwood Academic Publishers 1996:199-208.

Wa Thiong'o N. Moving the centre: The struggle for cultural freedoms. Nairobi: East African Educational Publishers, 1993a.

Wa Thiong'o N. The universality of local knowledge. In: Wa Thiong'o N. Moving the centre: The struggle for cultural freedoms. Nairobi: East African Educational Publishers, 1993b.

5
Comparing general health related quality of life (HRQoL) questionnaires; EuroQol, Sickness Impact Profile and Rosser Index

Stefan Björk and Ulf Persson

5.1 INTRODUCTION

In this paper differences and similarities between 3 commonly used HRQoL questionnaires will be the subject of a general discussion. We will use data from two different studies: one study on hip-joint replacement patients and one study on non-fatal traffic accidents.

Data from a study of total hip-replacement (Albinsson *et al*, 1992) and a comment on this data (Björk *et al*, 1992) as well as data from a study of non-fatal traffic accidents (Persson, 1992) are used. The paper concentrates on discussing possible explanations for differences between the questionnaires. These can refer to choices of dimensions and items to be included in the questionnaire as well as to weights attached to the items and dimensions used in the questionnaires.

5.2 PRESENTATION OF EUROQOL, SICKNESS IMPACT PROFILE AND ROSSER INDEX

We will only give a brief presentation of the 3 generic HRQoL questionnaires in this chapter, as they are considered public property.

EuroQol is a general HRQoL questionnaire (EuroQol Group, 1990). Since the start of the EuroQol Group in 1987, a number of versions have have been developed. As from 1993, 5 dimensions are included in the questionnaire, each containing 3 items. In the version used in the total hip replacement study, a version with 6 dimensions was used: mobility, self-care, usual activity, social relationships, pain and anxiety/depression. Usual activity, social relationships and anxiety/depression included 2 items and the other dimensions included 3 items. In addition to the dimensions, a thermometer with the endpoints 'best imaginable health state' and 'worst imaginable health state' was used. This thermometer rated the respondent's health state at the time he/she responded to the questionnaire. The respondent was also asked whether his/her state of health was worse, better or unchanged at the time of filling in the questionnaire compared to his/her health state during the last 12 months. The EuroQol questionnaire is spread over 2 pages and its results can be presented as an index or dimension by dimension.

P. Kind et al. (eds.), EQ-5D concepts and methods, 53–62.

The Sickness Impact Profile (SIP) includes 12 dimensions and 136 items (McDowell and Newell, 1987). The numbers of items in each dimension range from 7 to 23. The dimensions are: ambulation, mobility, body care and movement, social interaction, communication, alertness behaviour, emotional behaviour, sleep and rest, eating, work, household management, and recreation and pastimes. It is also possible to present the results in 3 dimensions (wherein the above-mentioned dimensions are included), as well as 1 overall score.

The Rosser Index is presented as a matrix comprising disability and distress (Rosser and Kind, 1987). However, a 3-dimensional version of the Rosser Index is now available where the third dimension is pain. Eight levels of disability and 4 levels of distress are included. The distress levels are: no distress, mild, moderate and severe distress. The disability levels are: 1/ No disability. 2/ Slight social disability. 3/ Severe social disability and/or slight impairment of performance at work. Able to do all housework except very heavy tasks. 4/ Choice of work or performance at work very severely limited. Housewives and old people able to do light housework only but able to go out shopping. 5/ Unable to undertake any paid employment. Unable to continue any education. Old people confined to home except for escorted outings and short walks and unable to go shopping. Housewives able only to perform a few simple tasks. 6/ Confined to chair or to wheel-chair or able to move around in the home only with support from an assistant. 7/ Confined to bed. 8/ Unconscious. The results of the Rosser Index are presented as an index.

5.3 DATA ON TOTAL HIP-REPLACEMENT

This section will present an investigation of health changes for patients who have undergone total hip-replacement surgery. On two occasions, measurements were made based on the EuroQol, SIP, and the Rosser Index. A 6-dimensional version of the EuroQol was used and the 2-dimensional version of the Rosser index. We will only briefly report the results expressed as index numbers. We will present the change between time point 1, i.e. before the operation, and time point 2, i.e. 6 months after the operation. We will report partly on the entire group, partly on each individual. This report includes 73 individuals in total (please note that the numbering in Table 5.2 represents individual numbers where non-responses are not included).

Table 5.1 Comparison of the index change before and after operation, for SIP, Rosser and EuroQol

	Comparison		Comparison		Comparison	
	SIP	Rosser	SIP	EuroQol	Rosser	EuroQol
Mean value	0.0639	0.0689	0.0662	0.1943	0.0709	0.1958
Standard deviation	0.070	0.070	0.067	0.195	0.071	0.194
Number of cases	72	72	68	68	69	69
P value T test	0.545		0.000		0.000	
P value Wilcoxon test	0.7168		0.000		0.000	

As can be seen from Table 5.1, the group's health has increased as a whole, over the 3 questionnaires. EuroQol showed the biggest increase in health, by almost 20%, compared with an SIP increase of aproximately 6%, and the Rosser Index by approximately 7%.

Table 5.2 Changes in health states per individual before and after hip joint surgery measured by EuroQol, SIP, and the Rosser Index

Individual number	SIP	Rosser	EuroQol	Individual number	SIP	Rosser	EuroQol
1	.10	.08	.	41	.03	-.04	-.20
2	.04	.03	.	42	.19	.09	.30
3	.05	.03	.10	43	.05	.09	.55
4	.08	.02	.13	45	.02	.04	.03
5	.13	.04	.03	46	.04	.03	.13
6	.04	.02	.14	47	.11	.12	.10
7	.09	.09	.45	48	.06	.04	.25
8	.05	.09	.10	49	.05	.01	.10
9	.07	.13	.30	50	.21	.12	.25
10	.04	.13	.60	51	.07	.03	.15
11	-.02	.12	-.10	52	.06	.04	.40
12	.16	.05	.30	53	.02	.04	.50
13	.02	.03	.20	54	.26	.26	.30
14	.07	.04	.30	55	.06	.04	.50
15	.00	.00	.08	56	-.02	.12	.45
16	.06	.04	.15	57	-.10	.00	.00
17	.20	.31	.20	58	.05	.01	.10
18	-.07	.09	-.10	59	.10	.07	.35

Table 5.2 Changes in health states per individual before and after hip joint surgery measured by EuroQol, SIP, and the Rosser Index (Continued)

Individual number	SIP	Rosser	EuroQol	Individual number	SIP	Rosser	EuroQol
19	.11	.12	.20	60	.05	.03	-.06
20	.09	.00	-.35	61	.07	.04	.30
21	.15	.07	.45	71	.08	.12	.64
22	.07	.12	.20	72	.09	.04	.30
23	.06	.04	.20	73	.02	.02	.00
24	.05	.06	.10	74	.04	.06	.10
26	.04	.04	.20	76	.07	.30	.20
27	.06	.06	.45	77	.	.08	.30
28	.08	.28	.55	78	.03	.	.
29	.07	.06	-.12	79	.09	.04	.24
30	-.17	-.03	-.15	80	.03	.07	.15
31	.23	.26	.10	81	- .13	.01	.
32	.14	.09	.09	82	.08	.06	.10
33	.08	.10	.00	83	.04	.04	.15
34	.10	.04	.30	84	.09	.03	.
35	.14	.04	.20	85	.05	.08	.30
36	.00	.03	.35	86	.05	.01	.10
37	.04	.07	.38	87	.05	.03	.00
40	.07	.02	.25	88	.05	.06	.15

At an individual level, there were differences between the individuals as well as between different questionnaires regarding the same individual. According to 2 of the questionnaires, 7 individuals have increased their health while they have reduced their health according to the third questionnaire (e.g. individual 11 in Table 5.2). There are differences regarding the same individual of as much as 56 percentage units depending on which questionnaire we focus. There are also large variations in the results for different individuals, ranging from a decrease in health by 35% to an increase by 64%.

5.4 DATA ON NON-FATAL TRAFFIC ACCIDENTS

This study was carried out as a prospective investigation of 1 year's new traffic casualties at 5 different casualty-receiving wards in Lund, Karlshamn, Karlskrona, Umeå. and Lidköping (all cities in Sweden). The investigation was unique in that it was intended to be a follow-up of the injuries 3 years after the accidents. The endpoint of the investigation was either death or full recovery with no further medical-care consumption due to the original traffic accident.

All individuals suffering from severe and slight injuries were asked to describe their health status on 4 different occasions. In connection with emergency care, the injured individuals received 2 questionnaires describing their health status 1 day and 1 week after the accident, respectively. Three weeks later, the individuals were asked to describe their health status 1 month after and just before the accident, respectively.

All individuals who were not fully recovered (but still alive) were followed up using additional questionnaires 6, 12, 24, and 36 months after the accident. Loss of health was measured by using the dimensions and levels defined in EuroQol and the Rosser Index. The 3-dimensional version of the Rosser Index was used, i.e. health was measured in terms of disability, distress and pain, and the weights were derived using the standard gamble (SG) technique. The 6-dimensional version of EuroQol was used.

The response rate was 60% for patients treated at Lund Hospital (so far, the only data analyzed). Table 5.3 shows the loss of health during 6 months after the accident for in-patient and out-patient traffic casualties at Lund Hospital measured by 3 different health indices.

Table 5.3 Average loss of health as a percentage of full health for in-patient and out-patient casualties at Lund Hospital 1 week, 1 month, and 6 months after accident, measured by 3 indices: EuroQol, Rosser Index, and Thermometer

		Percentage of loss of health measured by:								
		EuroQol			Rosser Index			thermometer		
	No. of pat.	1 week	1 month	6 months	1 week	1 month	6 months	1 week	1 month	6 months
in-patient casualties	15	49	43	27	21	17	10	40	31	17
out-patient casualties	79	31	18	7	13	8	4	25	15	8

At least 2 important points can be deduced from Table 5.3. Firstly, loss of health was greater for in-patient casualties at all points of time for all the 3 indices used compared to the out-patient casualties. Secondly, for all measurements the value of lost health was higher using the EuroQol index compared to the Rosser Index. The results on the thermometer lay somewhere in-between.

A subgroup of casualties consisting of 42 out-patients injured in bicycle accidents was analyzed in more detail. The average loss of health of these individuals is illustrated over a six month-period (Figure 5.1), assuming a constant rate of recovery between the measurement points.

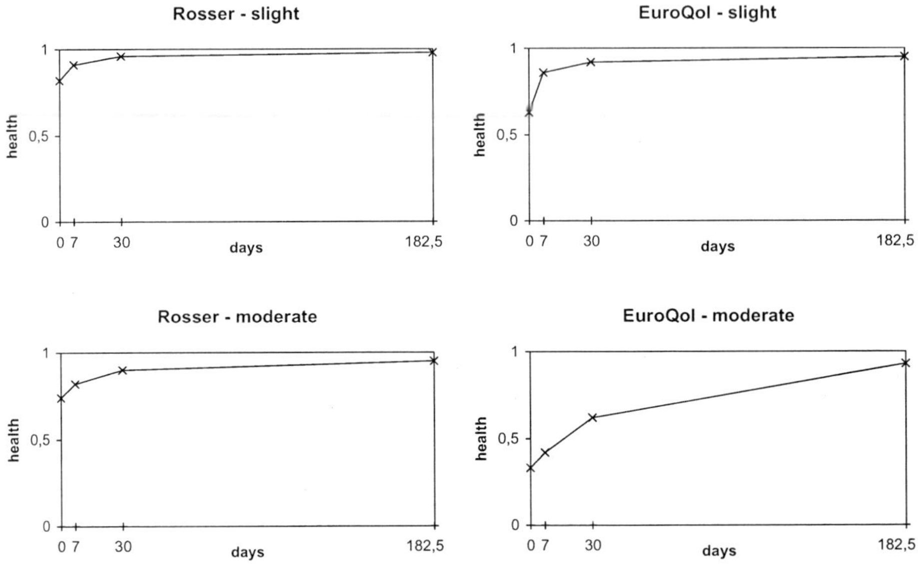

Figure 5.1 Average loss of health during the first 6 months after the accident for slight and moderate out-patient casualties measured by EuroQol and the Rosser Index.

The severity of a casualty is defined using the Injury Severity Score (ISS) with scores from 0 to 75. There were 21 casualties with light injuries, ISS (1-3), and 7 with moderate injuries. ISS (4-8). There were no out-patients injured with ISS 9 or above.

As can be seen from Figure 5.1, it is clear that the choice of health index is important for the results. The value of loss of health is about three times as high and about twice as high using the EuroQol index compared to the Rosser Index for moderate and light casualties, respectively.

5.5 DISCUSSION

The HRQoL instruments used in the present studies raise two interesting issues:

(i) What conclusions about changed HRQoL are supported by the results?
(ii) What are the explanations for the different results from the different questionnaires?

The first discussion will be empirical while the second will be methodological.

Empirical

Regarding the empirical issues concerning the study of total hip-replacement, the following may be observed: at a group level, all 3 questionnaires arrived at the same result - hip joint surgery leads to increased health. However, the different questionnaires showed increases in health of different magnitudes. The SIP and the Rosser Index yielded an increase in health of 6 to 7% while EuroQol yielded an increase of 20% (see Table 5.1). The explanation for this difference is to be found in the design of the 3 questionnaires.

At an individual level, there are also, of course, differences as to how the same individual responds to the different questionnaires. The biggest differences were seen for individual number 10 and individual number 71. Both had a difference of 56 percentage units between the SIP and EuroQol, where the bigger increase was registered by EuroQol. The explanation for this difference is also to be found in the design of the questionnaires.

Regarding the empirical issues concerning the non-fatal traffic accidents study, the following applies: it is evident that the measured values of loss of health for traffic casualties were at least twice as high using the EuroQol index compared with using Rosser's 3-dimensional index.

Methodological

The most plausible explanation for the differences between the different questionnaires employed in the total hip-replacement study is that they do not have the same sensitivity in detecting differences in hip joint patients in particular. This may be dependent on several factors. In designing a health or HRQoL questionnaire, one has to consider 3 issues (Björk, 1992). The standpoint made at this level should be guided by the overall objective of the questionnaire. The absence of such an objective affects the consistency of the questionnaire negatively.

(i) The first task is to choose the health states which are to be entered into the questionnaire.
(ii) The second one is to describe these health states.
(iii) The third task is to set the relative values of the different health states.

As far as the 3 questionnaires included in the present study are concerned, they differ on all the 3 points.

A possible explanation for the difference between the SIP and EuroQol is that the different questionnaires concentrate on different dimensions of health and quality of life. In the SIP, for example, there is no dimension of pain but in EuroQol there is. In fact, this dimension showed a large difference for the entire group in absolute numbers. The SIP concentrates on measuring behaviour, not feelings.

Individuals who have undergone total hip replacement experience a great increase in the dimension pain in particular. Generally, questionnaires which capture the dimensions where the measure undertaken is expected to have a beneficial effect (in the present case a hip joint operation) will, of course, also show the largest differences before and after the operations respectively.

Consequently, in this respect, EuroQol is more sensitive to changes than the SIP regarding patients who have undergone hip joint surgery.

The Rosser Index is designed for planning and evaluation within the health-care sector. Consequently, the overall objective is to help allocate health-care resources. This can be compared to the objective of the SIP, which is to measure behaviour, and the objective of EuroQol, which is to facilitate the collection of a common data set for reference purposes and to generate cross-national comparisons of health states (EuroQol Group, 1990). These different objectives of the 3 questionnaires have affected their design.

In the Rosser Index, 29 different health states are described with 2 dimensions: physical functional disability and distress/pain. Each of these has been assigned a weight - a value. The weight has been determined by 70 UK individuals (called respondents hereafter) who all had a connection to the health care system. The "magnitude estimation" method (Torrance, 1987) for producing these weights can briefly be described as follows. Out of the 29 different health states, 6 were presented to the respondents who were then asked to rank them. The ranking order defined which health state they prefered to be in and which health state they least prefered to be in, respectively. The other (23) health states were then entered on the ranking scale. Finally, a mean value of each of the health states was calculated. Every indication made by a patient stating that he or she was in this state was then adjusted according to the mean value. The weights produced in this way for the Rosser Index result in significant differences between some health states (see the double lines in the matrix, Table 5.4). A change between 2 health states will have a large effect (e.g. between 5C and 6D) while other changes will have considerably smaller effects (e.g. between 1A and 5C).

Table 5.4 Weightings according to the Rosser Index

		Distress/Pain			
		A	B	C	D
Functional disability		None	Mild	Moderate	Severe
I	None	1.000	0.995	0.990	0.967
II	Slight social disability	0.990	0.986	0.973	0.932
III	Social disability	0.980	0.972	0.956	0.912
IV	Work with difficulty	0.964	0.956	0.942	0.870
V	Unable to work	0.946	0.935	0.900	0.700
VI	Confined to chair	0.875	0.845	0.680	0.000
VII	Bed	0.677	0.564	0.000	-1.486
VIII	Unconscious	-1.028			

This implies that there is a 'step-like effect' built in to the 2 dimensional version of the Rosser Index which influences the degree of registered changes measured by this questionnaire. Large changes are registered around the 'steps', and small changes in health states which are not near the 'steps'.

The SIP consists of 136 items which means that there is a large number of possibilities for health state combinations. This can be compared with the Rosser Index which has 29 possible health states. A version of the same weighting procedure as was used by the Rosser Index has been applied to the SIP. Every SIP item has a weight which is correlated with all other items included in the questionnaire. Due to the multiplicity of items, each separate item is of less importance here than in the Rosser Index. The SIP contains more dimensions than the Rosser Index, though, which means that it describes the health states 'more comprehensively' than the Rosser Index. This might be one explanation of the differences in results between the 2 questionnaires at the individual level (Table 5.2).

EuroQol consists of 216 logically possible health states (based on the possible combinations of items) most of which are not realistic. The weighting of the items included in the individual's health state is based on the individual's own valuation of his/her own health. The 'step-like effect' of the Rosser Index as regards the distribution of weights between items does nor exist either in the SIP or in EuroQol. Their weightings of the health states are more evenly distributed. This is part of the explanation for the differences between the results of the 3 questionnaires.

The methodological differences between the 3 questionnaires, which have affected the results of the hip joint study, are partly the choice of dimensions, behavioural or psychological, partly the weighting of the items and the number of items included in the questionnaire.

Rosser's 3-dimensional index contains 7 levels of disability, 5 levels of distress, and 5 levels of pain. A standard gamble procedure was employed rather than the magnitude estimation procedure used in the previous 2-dimensional version. Rosser's 3-dimensional version does not contain the previous, step-like effect which results in high values of health changes despite small changes in health states.

However, it appeared that the values of the loss of health for non-fatal traffic injuries were at least twice as high as measured by EuroQol as when measured by Rosser's 3-dimensional index.

It seems that the choice of dimension to include in a health or quality of life questionnaire affects the way changes are measured to a great extent. As these choices are influenced by the overall aims of the questionnaire it is important to carefully scrutinize these aims before deciding which questionnaire to include in a study.

Presented at the EuroQol Plenary Meeting: Rotterdam, The Netherlands, 1993

5.6 REFERENCES

Albinsson G, Arnesson K, Fribeug H, Olsson K-E. Effects and costs of total hip-replacement in Karlskrona and Karlshamn. FoU Report. Lund: HSF (Council for Health Service Research), 1992.

Björk S. Metoder att värdera hälsa och livskvalitet (Methods for assigning values to health and quality of life). Socialmedicinsk tidskrift 1992;69(1):42-48.

Björk S, Althin R, Roos P. Livskvalitet vid total höftledsplastik, en kommentar till projektet "Effekter och kostnader av total höftledsplastik i Karlskrona och Karlsharmn". Mimeo: IHE, 1992.

EuroQol Group. A new facility for the measurement of health-related quality of life. Health Policy 1990;16:199-208.

McDowell I, Newell C. Measuring health. A guide to rating scales and questionnaires. Oxford, New York: Oxford University Press, 1987.

Persson U. Three economic approaches for valuing benefits of traffic safety measures. Lund: IHE, 1992.

Rosser R M, Kind P. A scale of valuations of states of illness. International Journal of Epidemiology 1978;7(4):347-358.

Torrance G W. Utility approach to measuring health-related quality of life. Journal of Chronic Disease 1987;40:593-600.

6
Influence of self-rated health and related variables on EuroQol-valuation of health states in a Spanish population

Xavier Badia, Esteve Fernandez and Andreu Segura

6.1 INTRODUCTION

In the last 5 years, much research has been conducted in order to obtain generic measures of health status comparable between different countries in a standardised way. In addition to the first steps made by the European group of the Nottingham Health Profile (Hunt *et al*, 1991), 2 more instruments are being currently adapted in European countries: the SF-36 (Aaronson, 1992) and the EuroQol (The EuroQol Group, 1990).

The objective of the instruments is different according to the background of the researchers. While the SF-36 is mainly focused on clinical decisions, the EuroQol is intended to aid policy decisions related to the allocation of resources. Thus, the approach to the valuation of the items and scales included in the instruments is different. The SF-36 uses a psychometric approach scoring the items by means of a Likert method, where the measure level of the attribute is the sum of responses to the questions for multiple items (Ware, 1992). The EuroQol has an economic approach that tries to obtain values by means of valuing holistic health states on a rating scale and the total score is the value assigned directly to a whole health state. Previous work of the EuroQol Group has tested the feasibility of the instrument by means of mailing questionnaires to random samples of the population. This research showed that no great differences exist among North-European cultures in valuation of health states included in the EuroQol (Essink-Bot, 1990; Nord, 1991; Brooks, 1991; Kind, 1991). Nevertheless, some methodological aspects of the EuroQol Instrument have been questioned (Car-Hill, 1992; EuroQol, 1992).

One of the most common problems in studies of the valuation of health states is the small number of raters used. In many cases this does not allow differences in health status values to be attributed to socio-demographic or health status characteristics. Several studies have found no differences in values assigned to health states attributable to socio-economic variables such as sex, age, socio-economic level or professional occupation (Carter, 1976; Rosser, 1978; Kaplan, 1976; Patrick, 1985; EuroQol Group, 1990). However, some authors have proved that medical knowledge, experience of illness, and the way that a health state is defined, labelled and presented, may influence the ratings of health states (Llewellyn-Thomas, 1984; Rosser, 1978;

P. Kind et al. (eds.), EQ-5D concepts and methods, 63–80.

Kaplan, 1976; Sackett and Torrance, 1978; Patrick, 1973). Recently some findings indicate that self-perceived health could also influence the ratings of health states (Kind, 1991; Brooks, 1991).

In Spain, 2 health profiles (the Nottingham Health Profile, and the Sickness Impact Profile) have been rigorously translated, the items rescaled by Spanish population samples, and their validity and reliability proved, showing equivalence with the original versions (Alonso, 1990; Badia and Alonso, 1993). But, until now, there have been no instruments suitable for use in cost-effectiveness studies which allow establishment of priorities within the broad spectrum of health interventions. Following the offer of the EuroQol Group (the EuroQol Group, 1990) to further assess the instrument, we chose it as a potential European instrument to produce a figure representing the quality of life that could be added to life years (Nord, 1992a).

The aim of this work was to test the feasibility of EuroQol and to analyse the influence of self-rated health and related variables on valuation of health states in a large sample of the Spanish population.

6.2 MATERIAL AND METHODS

For comparability purposes we used the revised EuroQol with 14 health states provided by 1 member of the EuroQol Group (P. Kind). The revised EuroQol Instrument is a self-administered generic measure of health status which contains 5 dimensions (mobility, self-care, usual activities, pain/discomfort and anxiety/depression) each with 3 items describing 3 different levels of function.

In the process of translating the Spanish version, we used 2 bilingual translators who produced 2 Spanish versions. These versions were back translated into English by 2 different bilingual speakers. The back translations were then evaluated by the translators and the research team. The semantic and conceptual equivalence was satisfactory (Brislin, 1973). Table 6.1 shows the dual English-Spanish layout.

Following a similar methodology developed by the EuroQol Group (1990) we obtained the values of the health states (a health state is a combination of 1 item from each of the 5 dimensions). Fourteen different health states (of 243 possible combinations) were included in the study. The health states were rated between 0 ('worst imaginable health state') and 100 ('best imaginable health state') on a visual analogue scale (VAS).

Table 6.1 Layout of the English and Spanish EuroQol

Mobility (Movilidad)

I have no problems in walking about
No tengo problemas para caminar

I have some problems in walking about
Tengo algunos problemas para caminar

I am confined to bed
Estoy siempre en la cama

Self-Care (Cuidado-Personal)

I have no problems with self-care
No tengo Droblemas con el cuidado personal

I have some problems washing or dressing myself
Tengo algunos problemas para lavarme o vestirme solo

I am unable to wash or dress myself
Soy incapaz de lavarme o vestirme solo

Usual Activities (Actividades Cotidianas)

I have no problems with performing my usual activities
No tengo problemas para realizar mis actividades cotidianas

I have some problems with performing my usual activities
Tengo algunos problemas para realizar mis actividades cotidianas

I am unable to perform my usual activities
Soy incapaz de realizar mis actividades cotidianas

Pain/Discomfort (Dolor/Malestar)

I have no pain or discomfort
No tengo dolor o malestar

I have moderate pain or discomfort
Tengo moderado dolor o malestar

I have extreme pain or discomfort
Tengo extremo dolor o malestar

Anxiety/Depression (Ansiedad/Depresión)

I am not anxious or depressed
No estoy ansioso o deprimido

I am moderately anxious or depressed
Estoy moderadamente ansioso o deprimido

I am extremely anxious or depressed
Estoy extremadamente ansioso o deprimido

A questionnaire was designed consisting of 5 pages. The first page included socio-demographic information and the self-descriptive part of the EuroQol Instrument. Individuals were required to mark the level of each dimension that they believed applied to them. On the second page, individuals were asked to: 1) score their own health on a VAS ranging from 0 to 100; 2) value 8 health states on a VAS ranging from 0 ('worst imaginable health state') to 100 ('best imaginable health state') by drawing a line from each health state to a point on the scale. On the third page, individuals valued 6 other health states; the best health state (11111) and the worst health state (33333) were repeated to check consistency in the ratings. On the fourth page the respondents were invited to go back to the second and third pages to mark the state "dead" on the VAS. On the fifth page, there were questions about level of education, experience of illness, experience of questionnaires, degree of difficulty in the valuation task and an open space to write opinions.

To test the feasibility of the questionnaire and especially the valuation task, we carried out a pilot study comprising 10 patients and 10 healthy people who attended a centre for disabled people. People with low socio-cultural levels were not able to fully understand the task of valuation of the states (50% of the sample). On the other hand, no-one had any difficulty in filling in the self-rating part of the EuroQol. The results of the pilot study and the low rates of response in postal surveys in Spain (Soriano, 1992), led us to consider alternative approaches to random sampling by mailed questionnaire.

We used a quota sampling method (Abrahamson, 1990) according to the following variables of stratification: gender (50% female); age (16-45, 50%; 46-60, 30%; > 60, 20%); occupational class (Domingo and Marcos, 1989) (classes I to III, 40%; classes IVV, 60%); and patient/non patient status (patients, 40%; non patients, 60%). We considered as a "patient" any person attending for a medical consultation due to an acute illness in the previous 7 days without prescription or due to a chronic illness in the previous 3 months; this included a request for medication for chronic pathology. A "non patient" was considered to be any person asking for prescriptions for a family member, asking about a family member's health, requesting a family member's illness certificate or attending a consultation for other administrative reasons.

Sample size was fixed at 600 valid questionnaires in order to detect differences between means of health states scores with a type I error of 1% and a statistical power of 90%.

The study was carried out in a Primary Health Care Centre in l'Hospitalet del Llobregat (Barcelona). In order to assign the potential respondents to a particular quota, the doctors involved in the study filled in a form with socio-demographic information obtained orally from potential candidates. Afterwards the doctor proposed participation in the study and, if the individual agreed to participate, he or she was sent to an adjacent room to perform the valuation task under the supervision of a trained nurse. Individuals who did not understand the task were substituted (12% of the sample) by another person in the same quota. The criteria used by the research team to decide such substitutions were: 1) large inconsistencies in rating health states (10%) ranking a determined health state in a non-logical way (e.g. 22213 valued higher than 11211), and 2) omission (2%) of valuation of 1 or more health states.

The mean, standard deviation and median of health states ratings were computed. Since ratings of health states for a given construct are assumed to be normally distributed, we compared average health state scores by means of Student's t-test and one-way analysis of variance when appropriate (Armitage, 1987). The chi-square test was performed to assess the relationship between socio-demographic characteristics and health state variables. Furthermore, multiple linear regression was used to control for confounding factors and to determine partial effects (Kleinbaum *et al*, 1988). The significance level was established at 0.01.

6.3 RESULTS

The average self-rated overall health status of the study population on the VAS was 76 (median 80) and ranged between 10 and 100. Tables 6.2 and 6.3 show the relationships of socio-demographic and health-related variables with self-rated overall health. No differences were found in self-rated overall health status between sex and occupational class. A pattern of decreasing ratings with increasing age was seen. Individuals with intermediate-university level of education rated their health higher than the group with only primary studies ($p < 0.001$), as did individuals who had no difficulty in carrying out the valuation task ($p < 0.001$). Individuals with some kind of experience of illness rated self-perceived overall health lower ($p < 0.001$) (Table 6.3). Individuals who described themselves as being in state 11111 rated their overall self-perceived health better than those in another health state ($p < 0.001$). No differences were found between patients/non patients.

When all the above variables were considered simultaneously in a multivariate analysis, age, experience of illness, degree of difficulty of the valuation task and self-described state 11111 were associated with self-rated overall health. Since only 15 individuals in the sample had previous experience of questionnaires, this variable was not used in the analysis.

Table 6.2 Self-rated overall health status by socio-demographic variables

	N	(%)	Mean	(SD)	Median	p	*
All respondents	600	(100)	76.1	(16.6)	80		
Gender							
Males	300	(50.0)	76.6	(15.5)	80		
Females	300	(50.0)	75.7	(17.7)	80	0.518	
Age (years)							
16-30	185	(30.8)	86.9	(11.1)	90		
31-45	115	(19,2)	80.9	(12.4)	80		
46-60	180	(30.0)	73.5	(14.2)	75		
61-75	114	(19.0)	59.1	(15.7)	60		
> 76	6	(1.0)	55.0	(15.7)	52	< 0.001	**
60 yrs	480	(80.0)	80.4	(13.9)	70		
> 60 yrs	120	(20.0)	58.9	(15.6)	60	< 0.001	
Occupational Class							
I-III	240	(40.0)	75.7	(17.3)			
IV-V	360	(60.0)	76.3	(16.3)		0.718	
Level of education #							
Primary school	335	(56.2)	71.3	(17.3)	70		
High School-Univ	261	(43.8)	82.7	(13.1)	85	< 0.001	
Degree of difficulty in the task							
Difficult	398	(66.4)	74.0	(17.6)	80		
Not difficult	201	(33.6)	80.5	(13.5)	80	< 0.001	

* Student's t-test

** One way analysis of variance

SD Standard deviation

\# Four missing values

Table 6.3 Self-rated overall health status by health-related variables

	N	(%)	Mean	(SD)	Median	p*
Patient/non patient						
Patient	240	(40.0)	76.2	(17.1)	80	
Non patient	360	(60.0)	76.1	(16.4)	80	0.937
Respondent's own experience of illness $						
Yes	70	(11.8)	56.5	(19.1)	50	
No	525	(88.2)	78.9	(14.4)	80	< 0.001
Respondent' s experience of illness in family						
Yes	212	(35.5)	68.1	(17.1)	70	
No	385	(64.5)	80.6	(14.7)	85	< 0.001
Respondent's experience in others &						
Yes	60	(10.1)	79.0	(16.0)	80	
No	534	(89.9)	75.9	(16.7)	80	0.167
Some experience of illness						
Yes	258	(43.0)	68.6	(18.0)	70	
No	342	(57.0)	81.8	(12.9)	85	< 0.001
Self-declared health state						
11111	310	(51.7)	86.5	(9.4)	90	
Other	290	(48.3)	65.0	(15.6)	70	< 0.001

* Student's t-test
$ Five missing values
# Three missing values
& Six missing values

The mean, standard deviations and median valuations of the 16 states of EuroQol are presented in Table 6.4. A consistent pattern between the states and the ratings is present. No differences were found between the repeated states (11111 and 33333). The standard deviations were greater in the intermediate states.

The valuation of the health states according to self-rated overall health is shown in Table 6.5. No clear differences were found according to self-rated health among the majority of health states. However, individuals rating perceived health higher rated states 22211 and 33321 higher ($p < 0.01$ in all cases), and 22322 and 'dead' somewhat lower.

Table 6.4 Average scores for the EuroQol Spanish study (n = 600)

Health state	Mean	SD	Median
11111	98.3	5.0	100
11111 R	98.6	4.7	100
11121	76.6	10.6	80
11112	75.8	10.9	80
21111	72.0	10.4	75
11211	70.6	10.9	70
11122	53.9	9.6	55
12111	52.6	10.7	50
21232	35.6	9.8	35
22322	22.3	10.5	30
22233	20.9	7.8	20
32211	12.7	12.1	10
33321	8.3	8.0	5
Dead-1	6.6	5.7	8
Dead-2	7.4	6.1	9
Unconscious	2.0	4.0	0
32333	2.3	4.5	0
33333 R	2.5	5.4	0

Table 6.5 Ratings of health states by self-rated overall health

	< 50 (n = 80)		51-75 (n = 178)		76-100 (n = 342)		
	Mean Median	(SD)	Mean Median	(SD)	Mean Median	(SD)	p*
11111	98.6	(5.3)	97.7	(6.2)	98.4	(4.1)	0.231
	100.0		100.0		100.0		
11111 R	98.8	(4.5)	98.1	(5.7)	98.7	(4.0)	0.299
	100.0		100.0		100.0		
11121	77.2	(11.9)	75.9	(10.7)	76.7	(10.2)	0.588
	80.0		80.0		80.0		
11112	76.2	(9.8)	75.1	(12.0)	76.1	(10.4)	0.575
	80.0		80.0		80.0		
21111	73.4	(9.7)	72.2	(8.6)	71.5	(11.4)	0.355
	75.0		75.0		74.0		
11211	72.4	(10.2)	70.5	(10.8)	70.3	(11.0)	0.293
	75.0		70.0		70.0		
11122	53.7	(8.9)	54.4	(9.2)	53.7	(9.9)	0.756
	55.0		55.0		55.0		
12111	53.2	(11.6)	51.9	(9.0)	52.8	(11.3)	0.583
	50.0		50.0		50.0		
21232	36.4	(10.2)	34.8	(9.4)	53.7	(9.9)	0.444
	35.0		35.0		35.0		
22322	34.8	(11.6)	33.5	(8.8)	31.1	(10.8)	0.002
	35.0		35.0		30.0		
22233	21.7	(7.5)	20.8	(7.8)	20.7	(7.8)	0.581
	20.0		20.0		20.0		
32211	9.4	(10.3)	11.5	(9.8)	14.1	(13.3)	0.002
	5.0		10.0		10.0		
33321	6.1	(6.0)	8.3	(7.7)	8.7	(8.4)	0.027
	5.0		5.0		5.0		
Dead-1	7.5	(6.7)	7.5	(5.2)	5.9	(5.6)	0.002
	8.0		8.0		6.0		
Dead-2	8.3	(7.0)	8.2	(5.5)	6.8	(6.1)	0.014
	10.0		10.0		8.0		
Unconscious	2.1	(6.7)	2.3	(5.9)	2.7	(6.4)	0.638
	0.0		0.0		0.0		
33333	1.7	(3.9)	2.1	(4.0)	2.6	(4.8)	0.199
	0.0		0.0		0.0		
32333 R	1.8	(3.5)	3.0	(4.2)	2.9	(6.1)	0.065
	0.0		0.0		0.0		

* One way analysis of variance

SD Standard deviation

Further analyses were conducted to assess the potential relationship between other variables and the valuation of health states, focusing on socio-demographic and health variables. Individuals over 60 or with low levels of education rated most of the states slightly higher. In most of the states, the differences reached the 1% level of statistical significance (Tables 6.6 and 6.7), although the magnitude of the observed differences were small. The level of education was related to the degree of understanding the valuation task. 76% of the individuals with low levels of education found the task difficult or very difficult compared with 60% of individuals with intermediate or high levels of education ($p < 0.001$). Table 6.8 shows the values of health states by degree of difficulty of the task. The EuroQol health state (derived from the 5 dimensions) was not strongly associated with the valuation of health states (Table 6.9).

Table 6.6 Ratings of health states by age

	≤ 60 years (n=480)		> 60 years (n=120)		
	Mean	(SD)	Mean	(SD)	p*
11111	98.1	(5.2)	99.1	(4.1)	0.013
11111 R	98.4	(5.0)	99.4	(3.2)	0.006
11121	76.4	(10.7)	77.2	(10.5)	0.472
11112	73.4	(11.1)	77.7	(9.9)	0.037
21111	71.3	(10.9)	74.6	(7.9)	< 0.001
11211	70.2	(11.2)	72.4	(9.4)	0.025
11122	54.0	(10.0)	53.7	(7.9)	0.775
12111	52.8	(10.9)	51.6	(9.8)	0.246
21232	35.2	(10.1)	37.3	(8.7)	0.019
22322	31.8	(10.5)	34.3	(9.9)	0.017
22233	20.5	(7.9)	22.1	(7.5)	0.045
32211	13.4	(12.6)	10.0	(9.9)	0.002
33321	8.7	(8.5)	6.3	(5.1)	< 0.001
Dead-1	6.3	(5.9)	7.9	(5.0)	0.002
Dead-2	7.0	(6.2)	8.9	(5.5)	0.003
Unconscious	2.8	(6.8)	1.4	(3.5)	0.002
33333	2.4	(4.5)	2.0	(4.4)	0.377
33333 R	2.7	(5.5)	1.8	(4.7)	0.090

* Student's t-test

Table 6.7 Ratings of health states by level of education

	Primary school (n = 335)		High School/ University (n = 261)		
	Mean	(SD)	Mean	(SD)	p*
11111	98.8	(4.1)	97.6	(5.9)	0.004
11111 R	99.2	(3.3)	97.8	(6.0)	0.001
11121	77.6	(9.6)	75.1	(11.7)	0.006
11112	76.8	(9.8)	74.4	(12.0)	0.008
21111	72.6	(10.7)	71.2	(10.2)	0.117
11211	71.8	(9.9)	69.3	(12.0)	0.007
11122	54.0	(8.7)	53.8	(10.7)	0.777
12111	51.4	(10.0)	54.2	(11.4)	0.002
21232	35.8	(9.9)	35.3	(9.8)	0.513
22322	33.4	(9.6)	30.8	(11.3)	0.003
22233	21.3	(7.9)	20.4	(7.8)	0.153
32231	10.4	(9.3)	15.9	(14.5)	< 0.001
33321	6.9	(5.9)	10.1	(9.8)	< 0.001
Dead-1	6.9	(5.3)	6.2	(6.3)	0.120
Dead-2	7.8	(5.7)	6.9	(6.6)	0.087
Unconscious	2.1	(5.1)	3.1	(7.6)	0.051
33333	2.0	(4.1)	2.7	(5.0)	0.082
33333 R	2.3	(5.6)	2.8	(5.0)	0.270

* Student's t-test

Table 6.8 Ratings of health states by degree of difficulty of the task

	Very Difficult Difficult (n = 398)		Easy Very Easy (n = 201)		
	Mean	(SD)	Mean	(SD)	p*
11111	98.8	(3.8)	97.1	(6.6)	0.001
11111 R	99.2	(2.9)	97.3	(6.8)	< 0.001
11121	77.7	(9.5)	74.2	(12.2)	< 0.001
11112	77.0	(9.7)	73.4	(12.5)	< 0.001
21111	73.8	(9.0)	68.4	(11.9)	< 0.001
11211	71.9	(10.1)	68.0	(12.0)	< 0.001
11122	53.7	(9.0)	54.3	(10.7)	0.054
12111	52.0	(9.6)	53.4	(12.6)	0.109
21232	35.2	(9.2)	36.2	(10.9)	0.289
22322	33.9	(8.9)	29.1	(3.2.3)	< 0.001
22223	20.6	(7.5)	21.2	(8.4)	0.394
32211	10.4	(9.5)	17.3	(15.1)	< 0.001
33321	6.9	(6.3)	10.9	(10.0)	< 0.001
Dead-1	6.9	(5.6)	6.0	(5.9)	0.106
Dead-2	7.8	(6.1)	6.7	(6.1)	0.030
Unconscious	2.1	(6.1)	3.3	(6.8)	0.027
33333	1.7	(3.9)	3.3	(5.4)	< 0.001
33333 R	1.8	(3.9)	3.7	(7.2)	0.001

* Student's t-test

Table 6.9 Ratings of health states by respondent's health state

	Health state 11111 (n = 310)		Rest of health states declared (n = 290)		
	Mean	(SD)	Mean	(SD)	p*
11111	98.0	(5.0)	98.5	(5.0)	0.295
11111 R	98.4	(4.8)	98.7	(4.5)	0.447
11121	76.0	(11.0)	77.1	(10.1)	0.150
11112	75.0	(11.7)	76.8	(10.0)	0.041
21111	71.3	(10.7)	72.7	(10.1)	0.094
11211	70.0	(11.4)	71.2	(10.3)	0.182
11122	52.6	(9.8)	55.3	(9.2)	0.001
12111	52.0	(10.8)	53.2	(10.6)	0.186
21232	34.7	(10.1)	36.4	(9.4)	0.031
22322	31.2	(10.3)	33.5	(10.5)	0.006
22233	20.3	(7.6)	2114	(8.0)	0.075
32211	13.0	(12.1)	12.4	(12.2)	0.553
33321	8.8	(8.7)	7.7	(7.0)	0.079
Dead-1	5.9	(5.7)	7.3	(5.7)	0.003
Dead-2	6.6	(6.0)	8.2	(6.1)	0.001
Unconscious	2.7	(6.4)	2.3	(6.3)	0.404
33333	2.3	(4.3)	2.3	(4.7)	0.941
33333 R	2.6	(5.4)	2.3	(5.3)	0.484

* Student's t-test

Sex, occupational class, patient/non patient status and previous experience of illness did not have a relevant influence (not more than 2 health states per variable were statistically different) in ratings of health states (data not shown).

The multivariate analysis carried out for each of 16 health states showed that the degree of difficulty of the task and age were associated with most of the health states valued. In addition to the previous variables, educational level and experience of illness were also associated for states 11111, 33321 and 32211.

6.4 DISCUSSION

There were some problems with the feasibility of EuroQol in the Spanish population. The instrument was administered to a sample of 600 individuals from the general population recruited through a quota sampling method. This was chosen due to the low rates of response in postal surveys in Spain, as well as difficulty in carrying out the valuation task. The difficulty of understanding the valuation task was shown in the pilot study and confirmed in the present study (most individuals rated the task of valuation as difficult and only 15 out of the 600 individuals had previous experience in filling out questionnaires). On the other hand, bivariate and multivariate analysis showed that age, level of education, experience of illness and especially the degree of difficulty of the valuation task was associated with the valuation of health states. Nevertheless, the differences were small and no consistent pattern were seen in the meaning or direction of these differences.

One of the weaknesses observed in previous studies which aimed to achieve values of health states was the small number of raters used. The maximum size of 10 selected studies of valuation of health states reviewed recently by Nord (1992b) was 121 raters, and most studies employed "selected" health-care personnel as raters. In this review, only 1 study was carried out in the general population (Nord, 1991) and 1 study with patients (Llewellyn-Thomas, 1984). As a result of this limitation, it is uncertain whether socio-demographic or perceived health variables influence the valuation of health states.

In addition, the low rate of response obtained with postal questionnaires may be a source of bias. All previous EuroQol studies have used a postal questionnaire in a representative sample of the population and low response rates were obtained. Moreover, the usable responses of the studies for analysis were even lower (37% in The Netherlands, 23% in the UK and 21% in Sweden) (EuroQol Group, 1990). Older people and individuals with low levels of education were also under-represented in the samples (Essink-Bot, 1990; Kind, 1991). Furthermore, while in the North-European EuroQol studies approximately 60% of respondents described the task as easy or very easy, 66.3% of the Spanish respondents rated it as difficult or very difficult. This might be explained by selection bias: the questionnaires were only returned by the individuals who understood (or believed they understood) the valuation task while those considering it to be difficult did not return the questionnaires.

In the present study we have tried to obtain values from a large sample of the general population, previously determining the characteristics of the sample (quota sampling). Although this approach did not provide a representative sample of the general population, it served to guarantee the presence of respondents with different characteristics thus trying to avoid non-response bias. So, a strength of this study is the large number and wide spectrum (including patients) of respondents included.

We found significant differences in self-rated overall health when respondents were grouped according to the remaining variables. As expected, the main differences were found by age, level of education, experience of illness and self-described health state. We did not find differences according to sex or occupational class or patient/non patient status or self-perceived overall health. A possible explanation might be the low level of severity of disease of the patients included in this study (e.g. hypertension). Control for these factors was not possible since the level of severity of the disease was not requested.

The rank order of health states scored followed a logical pattern and incongruences were not found. Individuals considered a drop in the level of health on self-care, usual activities and mobility to be more important than pain/discomfort or anxiety/depression. This would indicate that an impairment in a self-care dimension is considered as more relevant than in pain, which is rated lower (76 versus 52 respectively). Thus the different contribution of each dimension in the average score of a determined health state should be taken into account in future research.

As previously observed by other authors, extreme forms of combined disability and distress lead to lower values, even values worse than death (Rosser, 1978; Kaplan, 1976; EuroQol Group, 1990). This concern has been discussed elsewhere and remains an open debate (Sintonen, 1981).

The influence of socio-demographic and health variables in valuation of health states is controversial. Froberg (1989) states that "the literature on rater differences suggests that while age and experience with health state being rated (not general health status) may influence raters' valuations, the effects of most other demographic and experiental/medical variables are small or inexistent".

In the Spanish sample studied, self-rated overall health, self-rated health state, age, and level of education had a different degree of influence on values of health states. While differences by age and level of education were found, fewer differences arose from self-rated health variables. Similar results were obtained by Sackett (1978) in 240 individuals from the general population. But the variable that had the greatest influence in the valuation of health states was the self-declared degree of difficulty of the task. Individuals who declared difficulty had a low socio-economic level, low level of education and were older ($p < 0.001$).

Few studies have explored the influence of self-rated health on valuation of health states. Llewellyn-Thomas *et al* (1984) found that self-rated health had no influence on a sample of 64 cancer patients. Churchill *et al* (1984) found no differences regarding past experience of hospitalization, serious illness, history of severe pain, or family history of serious illness. Recently, Kind (1990) and Brooks (1990) using the EuroQol in the general population found that people who rated their health better valued the “preferable” health states higher and the “bad” health states lower. In the present study, self-rated health states had significant differences in only 4 health state values. Individuals who described themselves as being in “perfect health” (state 11111) in the 5 dimensions of the instrument gave the 4 health states a lower score than the individuals who described themselves as having some problem in at least 1 dimension.

The results obtained suggest that to achieve values for health states from the general population suitable for application in policy decision-making we should be sure that the method employed is understood by the raters. Variations of health state values according to socio-demographic variables could be explained by the self-perceived difficulty of the required task. Thus stratification by socio-demographic variables is not important. This would be different if the goal were to obtain values from patients to be applied in clinical decision-making where such values would be influenced by the condition itself, the severity, and the prognosis of the condition (Torrance, 1987), thus sampling patients with selected characteristics would be necessary.

However, differences cannot be explained only by socio-demographic and health status characteristics. Further research concerning biases in judgement (Tversky, 1974) and the method used (VAS) is necessary to clarify their impact on health state values.

Presented at the EuroQol Plenary Meeting: Rotterdam, The Netherlands, 1993

6.5 REFERENCES

Aaronson N X, Acquadro C, Alonso J, Apolone G, Bucquet D, Bullinger M, Bungay K, Fukuhara S, Gandek B, Keller S, Razavi D, Sanson-Fisher R, Sullivan M, Wood-Dauphine S, Wagner A, Ware J E. International quality of life assessment (IQOLA) project. Quality of Life Research 1992;1:349-351.

Abrahamson J H. Survey methods in community medicine (4th ed). New York: Churchill-Livingstone, 1990:80.

Alonso J, Antó J M, Moreno C. The Spanish version of the Nottingham Health Profile: Translation and preliminary validity. Am J Public Health 1990;80:704-708.

Armitage P, Berry G. Statistical methods in medical research (2nd ed.). Oxford: Blackwell Scientific Publications, 1987.

Badia X, Alonso J. Adaptación de una medida de la disfunción relacionada con la enfermedad. La versión española del Sickness Impact Profile. Med Clin (Barc.) 1994;102(3):90-95.

Brislin R, Lowner W, Thorndike R. Cross cultural research methods. New York: Wiley and Sons, 1973;32-81.

Brooks R G, Jendleg S, Lindgren B, Persson U, Bjork S. Health related quality of life measurement. Results of the Swedish Questionnaire Exercise, Health Policy 1991;18:37-48.

Carr-Hill R A. A second opinion: Health related quality of life measurement- Euro style. Health Policy 1992;20:321-328.

Carter W B, Bobbit R A, Bergner M, Gibson B S. Validation of an interval scaling: The Sickness Impact Profile. Health Serv Res 1976;Winter:516-528.

Churchill D N, Mayan J, Torrance G W. Quality of life in end stage renal disease. Peritoneal Dialysis Bulletin 1984;4:20-23.

Domingo A, Marcos J. Propuesta de un indicador de la "clase social" basado en la ocupación. Gaceta Sanitaria 1989;10(3):320-326.

Essink-Bot M L, Bonsel G J, Van der Maas P J. Valuation of health states by the general public: Feasibility of a standardised measurement procedure. Social Science and Medicine 1990;31:1201-1206.

EuroQol Group. EuroQol - A new facility for the measurement of health related quality of life. Health Policy 1990;16:199-208.

EuroQol. A reply and reminder. Health Policy 1992;20:329-332.

Froberg D G, Kane R L. Methodology for measuring health-state preferences-III: Population and context effects. J Clin Epidemiol 1989;42(6):585-592.

Hunt S M, Alonso J, Bucquet D, Niero M, Wiklund I, McKenna S. Cross-cultural adaptation of health measures. Health Policy 1991;19:33-44.

Kaplan R M, Bush J W, Berry C. Health status: Types of validity and the index of well being. Health Ser Res 1976;11:478.

Kind P. Measuring valuations for health states: A survey of patients in general practice. Discussion Paper No. 76, Centre for Health Economics, University of York, 1991.

Kleinbaum DO, Kupper LI, Muller KE. Applied regression analysis and other multivariable methods. Boston: PWS-KENT Publishing Company, 1988.

LLewellyn-Thomas H, Sutherland H J, Tibshirani R, Ciampi A. Till J E, Boyd N F. Methodologic issues in obtaining values for health states. Med Care 1984; 22: 543-552.

Nord E. EuroQol health-related quality of life measurement, valuations of health states by the general public in Norway. Health Policy 1991;18:25-36.

Nord E. The use of EuroQol values in QALY calculations. In: Bjork S, editor. EuroQol Conference, Lund, October 1991: Proceedings, IHE Working Paper Institute of Health Economics, Lund, Sweden, 1992a.

Nord E. Methods for quality adjustment of life years. Soc Sci Med 1992b;34:559-569.

Patrick D, Bush J W, Chen M M. Toward an operational definition of health. Journal of Health and Social Behaviour 1973;14:6-23.

Patrick D, Sittampalam Y, Sommerville S, Carter W, Bergner M. A cross-cultural comparison of health status values. Am J Public Health 1985;75:1402-1407.

Rosser R, Kind P. A scale of valuations of states of illness: Is there a social consensus? Int J Epidemiol 1978;7:347.

Sackett D L, Torrance G W. The utility of different health states as perceived by the general public. J Chron Dis 1978;7:347-358.

Sintonen H. An approach to measuring and valuing health states. Soc Sci Med 1981;15C:55-65.

Soriano J B, Sabrià J, Sunyer J, Antó J M. Resposta a un qüestionari per correu o per telèfon. A propòsit de la prova pilot a Barcelona de l'Estudi Europeu d'Asma. Ann Med (Barc.) 1992;LXXVIII(6):149-153.

Torrance G W. Utility approach to measuring health related quality of life. J Chron Dis 1987;40(6):593-600.

Tversky A, Kahheman D. Judgement under uncertainty: heuristic and biases, Science 1974;185:1124-1131.

Ware J E. Donald Sherbourne C. The MOS 36-item short from health survey (SF-36). I. Conceptual framework and item selection. Med Care 1992;30(6):473-482.

7
Observations on one hundred students filling in the EuroQol questionnaire

Jan Busschbach, Dick Hessing and Frank de Charro

7.1 INTRODUCTION

The EuroQol Instrument measures HRQoL (EuroQol, 1990). The questionnaire was developed by the EuroQol Group, an international group of scientists working together in the field of measuring HRQoL. In developing the EuroQol, one of the ambitions was to make the questionnaire suitable for postal distribution. Hence, almost all research carried out using the EuroQol Instrument is by means of postal surveys. A disadvantage of this is that the researcher does not know how the subjects fill in the questionnaire. Of course, the investigator can ask some simple written questions and he/she can analyze the remarks in the margin, but observations and more complex questions are impossible. In order to address this issue, 100 students filled in the questionnaire while the first author was present, enabling him to make observations and asked questions afterwards.

Some of the specific research questions for this investigation were based on the regular scientific literature about the EuroQol Instrument (The EuroQol Group, 1990, 1991, 1992; Nord, 1991; Brooks, 1991; Carr-Hill, 1992; Essink-Bot, 1990). However, most of the questions were inspired by the Scientific Meetings of the EuroQol Group and the reports of the pilot studies that have been circulated within the Group. Some of these reports have been printed in scientific series published by research centres. An example of this literature is the EuroQol proceedings from Lund, Sweden edited by Björk (1992). However, most of the knowledge is still circulating in hard copy and is not publicly known. An attempt to collect this body of knowledge was undertaken by Nord in 1991. He gathered the findings and comments on the pilot studies and brought them together in the Index EuroQolus. Many of the research questions in this investigation are mentioned in EuroQolus, so it will serve as a reference for this chapter.

In the past, there has only been one attempt to carry out an observed administration of the EuroQol. This was undertaken by Ashby, Rushby and O'Hanlon in 1988. It was a small pilot study, in which the EuroQol questionaire was filled in by 16 members of the university staff at Brunel University, UK. The report of the pilot study is referenced in EuroQolus as Brunel 1, and contains one and a half pages of observations and comments by the subjects. Although the number of subjects was low and the reporting limited, the pilot study raised a number of important hypotheses about the way subjects fill in the questionnaire.

P. Kind et al. (eds.), EQ-5D concepts and methods, 81–90.

Because this investigation does not test just one hypothesis but a number of research questions, the structure of this chapter was adjusted. The methods section describes only the EuroQol Instrument itself and the general structure of the experiment. The hypotheses, method of testing, and the results are grouped by research question.

7.2 METHOD

The EuroQol Instrument.

The first description of the EuroQol Instrument was published in 1990 (EuroQol Group, 1990). Since this first article, the questionnaire has been changed. The version used in this investigation conforms to the modifications made at the EuroQol Conference in Lund, Sweden in 1991. The first page of the EuroQol contains general information about the purpose of the questionnaire. After the introduction, the subjects were asked which EuroQol health state they were in. The EuroQol health states are described according to 5 dimensions, each with 3 levels. The dimensions and levels are listed in Table 7.1.

Table 7.1 Dimensions, levels and the codes of the health states

Digit Place	Dimension	Code	Category
I	Mobility	1	No problems in walking about.
		2	Some problems in walking about.
		3	Confined to bed.
II	Self-Care	1	No problems with washing or dressing self
		2	Some problems with washing or dressing self
		3	Unable to wash or dress self
III	Usual Activities	1	No problems with performing usual activities (e.g. work, study, housework, family or leisure activities).
		2	Some problems with performing usual activities (e.g. work, study, housework, family or leisure activities).
		3	Unable to perform usual activities (e.g. work, study, housework, family or leisure activities).
IV	Pain / Discomfort	1	No pain or discomfort
		2	Moderate pain or discomfort
		3	Extreme pain or discomfort
V	Anxiety / Depression	1	Not anxious or depressed
		2	Moderately anxious or depressed
		3	Extremely anxious or depressed

A EuroQol health state can be described as a 5 digit code. The first digit represents the category of mobility, the second self-care, etc. For instance, the health state in figure 7.1 can be represented by the number 33321.

- Confined to bed.
- Unable to wash or dress self.
- Unable to perform usual activities (e.g. work, study, housework, family or leisure activities)
- Moderate pain or discomfort.
- Not anxious or depressed

Figure 7.1 EuroQol health state 33321

After the subjects classified themselves according to the EuroQol health state descriptive system, they indicated their own health on a vertical, calibrated scale, numbered from 0-100. The bottom of the scale was labelled 'the worse imaginable health state' and the top was labelled 'best imaginable health state'. After the instructions, the main task started. Two pages each with 8 health states were presented either side of the calibrated scale. On both pages, states 11111 and 33333 were repeated. The subjects were asked to draw lines from the health states to points on the scale which indicated how good or how bad the health states were, in their view.

Following this task, the subjects answered some written questions about their socio-economic status.

The subjects were not allowed to ask any questions about the questionnaire when they filled it in, but were told to follow the written instructions. Only when a student could not continue or the subject's responses indicated that the task was unclear, were additional spoken instructions given. After the students filled in the questionnaire, they were asked some verbal questions about the task. For example, one of the questions was: 'What would you have answered if the health state which was labelled unconscious had been labelled death?'.

Posters introducing the investigation were hung in the university's cafeteria at Erasmus University, The Netherlands. The poster advertised a 25 Guilder (US $17.00, September 1992) payment for participating in an interview concerning 'the assessment of health states', which would last for one and a half hours.

7.3 RESULTS

The subjects.

First a pilot study was set up with 10 subjects. A total of 105 students cooperated in the main investigation. The students had an average age of 22.70 years (SD 3.77) and 39% were female. Almost half of the students (48.6%) came from the faculty of Law, 16.2% from the faculty of Public Administration, 14.3% from the faculty of Economics, 11.4% from the faculty of Sociology and 9.5% from various other faculties. Every subject finished the questionnaire.

Table 7.2 The means and standard deviations of the health states

Health States	Mean	SD	Health States	Mean	SD
11111[a]	0.92	0.08	22233	0.26	0.13
11111[b]	0.91	0.09	33321	0.24	0.14
11211	0.75	0.13	22323	0.23	0.12
11121	0.70	0.13	Unconscious[c]	0.20	0.20
21111	0.69	0.14	Death[d]	0.12	0.22
11112	0.67	0.15	33333[b]	0.10	0.10
12111	0.61	0.16	33333[a]	0.09	0.10
11221	0.55	0.12	21232	0.35	0.13
32211	0.43	0.16	22233	0.26	0.13
21232	0.35	0.13			

a. State appearing at the first page of the EuroQol Visual Analogue Scale.
b. State appearing at the second page of the EuroQol Visual Analogue Scale.
c. Values between 0 and 100, N = 102.
d. Values between 0 and 100, N = 75.

The difficulty of the main valuation task

After the valuation of the EuroQol health states, the EuroQol Instrument asks the subject how difficult it was to fill in the questionnaire. One percent of the students said that it was very difficult, 36% fairly difficult, 65% fairly easy and 5% very easy. From these results it can be concluded that most of the subjects (70%) found it to be fairly easy to very easy to fill in the questionnaire. Similar results were found for the general public. For example in the investigation of Essink-Bot (1990), 57% of the general public found the postal questionnaire to be fairly easy to very easy to fill in. However, almost all authors reported that many mistakes were made. For example, in the investigation of Essink-Bot study, only 81 out of 112 questionnaires (72.3%) contained usable valuations of the health states on pages 5 and 6. From their observations in 1988, Ashby and her colleagues concluded that when respondents said that the questionnaire was rather easy, they referred to the whole questionnaire, including the easy questions at the beginning and end (EuroQolus, 7.4; Brunel, 1). In order to test this hypothesis, subjects were asked to indicate how difficult it was to value the health states, after reading the instructions. Only 41% answered that the task was fairly easy or very easy, so it appears that Ashby and her colleagues were correct.

The remarks that the subjects made after they finished the EuroQol gave further indications that the main task was difficult. In fact, most remarks made were about the valuation task. Sixteen of the 105 respondents said that it was hard to compare the 8 health states on 5 dimensions simultaneously. Ten subjects said almost the same by indicating that it was hard to be consistent. Fifteen students found it hard to picture the health states. In addition 6 students found the calibration of the scale too fine for such a complex task. It has been suggested that the task might be difficult because valuing health states causes emotional stress. This did not seem to be the case in the current study, because only one student made a remark about emotional stress.

Mistakes and the instructions.

Fifty-five percent of the students claimed that the instructions were clear. However, 71% of the students had to go back and forth between the instructions and the valuation task, which indicated that the instructions were not completely understood after one reading. But although the task seemed complicated, only a few serious mistakes were made. One of the most striking mistakes was the interpretation of the label 'best imaginable health state' located above the calibrated scale, and the interpretation of the instruction 'Remember, we want you to indicate how good or bad each of these states would be for a person like you.' Sixteen students thought that the aim was to indicate how well one could imagine being in the health states themselves. Of the 16 students who made this mistake initially, 7 corrected themselves after valuing a few states. The other 9 subjects continued and were corrected by the investigator. The scores of the subjects who made this mistake had a typical dichotomous distribution. Since most students have never been in a bad health state, they found it most difficult to imagine the bad health states. Therefore, all the bad states had extreme low values and the good health states had extreme high values. These dichotomous scores were also noted by Brooks in 1991. In order to avoid confusion about the word 'imaginable', it would perhaps be better to eliminate the word or to replace it with 'the best health state'.

Sintonen (EuroQolus 5.1 A; Sintonen, Helsinki, 6:4) noticed that some subjects started to draw lines from the dimensions (the sentences) of the health states, instead of from the health states as a whole. In this investigation 5 students started to do this. Three students corrected themselves, but 2 others had to be corrected by the investigator. When the students valued their own health states on page 3, 11 students did not draw a line from the box to the scale, but indicated the value in some other way. This mistake did not have very serious consequences, because the scores were still usable. However, it is an indication that the task is unfamiliar for many people. Afterwards, 7 subjects remarked that drawing lines was not very common and therefore caused confusion.

Students have better cognitive capacities than the general public. Hence, it is likely that the general public would have experienced more difficulties with the questionnaire than the students. On the other hand, it is reasonable to expect that problems encountered by students will also be present in the general public.

The 1 year period.

The instructions for the main valuation task read: 'When thinking about the health state imagine that it will last for 1 year. What happens after that is not known and should not be taken into account'. This instruction is important because the value of a health state is dependent on its duration. For instance, Sutherland (1982) found that the utility of a bad health state decreases after a certain duration, which she called the maximum endurable time. During Ashby's investigation in 1988, 18 of the 37 subjects forgot the instructions of the 1 year interval and thought about a chronic health state (EuroQolus 5.1 A and 5.1 E; Brunel, 1). In the present investigation, the subjects were asked which time interval they had in mind when they valued the health states. Table 7.3 gives the results.

Table 7.3 The actual time interval subjects used

Time interval	Number	%
One year	36	34.5
A chronic state	28	6.7
A period longer than 1 year, but not clearly defined	25	23.8
No time period in mind	8	7.6
Months	5	4.8
Days	2	1.9
Weeks	1	1.0

As can be seen from Table 7.3, only 34.5% of the subjects remembered the instruction about the 1 year time interval. Where the subjects forgot the instruction, they were most likely to believe that the states would be stable for a period of time longer than 1 year. Both Nord and Bonsel (EuroQolus 10.E; Bonsel/Bot, Rotterdam, EuroQolus 10:1 and 10.F; Nord, Oslo, 5:4) have suggested that the duration of 1 year would give problems with the valuation of death. Two subjects said that it was impossible to be dead for 1 year. However, there was no significant systematic relationship between the actual time interval used by the subjects and the value of death. A suggestion would be to drop the 1 year instruction and to work with chronic states.

The order of valuation.

A point that is often discussed is do the subjects employ a strategy, or do they simply fill in the questionnaire? This investigation provided an opportunity to observe the order of the valuations. Table 7.4 gives the results of these observations.

Table 7.4 The observed order of the valuations on pages 5 and 6

Order of filling in	page 5	page 6
First the left column, then the right column.	54.3%	53.3%
From left to right, like reading a book	14.3%	14.3%
No recognizable strategy	13.3%	14.3%
Makes a ranking first	8.6%	8.6%
Seeks the best or the worst first, then no recognizable strategy.	8.6%	8.6%

Only 7.6% of the subjects changed their strategy from pages 5 to 6, and 31.4% went back and forth between pages 5 and 6, in order to compare the valuations on both pages. From these results we concluded that only a minority uses a strategy. The majority just takes the task as it comes.

The influence of the depression dimension.

It has been suggested that the dimension depression and anxiety has a relatively high influence on the value of a health state, because this dimension could be seen as an interpretation of physical health (EuroQolus 5.5 B; Nord, Oslo, 6:2 and 13.E; Brunel, 1). This view has been supported by another observation of Ashby and her colleagues (EuroQolus 8.A; Brunel, 1). Some of their subjects said that it is impossible to be in a bad physical state without feeling depressed. In order to investigate this, the subjects were asked if they saw the psychological dimension as dependent or independent of the physical dimensions. From the sample, 48.6% saw these 2 dimensions as independent, 34.7% as dependent and 16.7% did not know. However, the values obtained by the independent subjects did not differ significantly from those of the dependent subjects (tested univariatly on all health states, T-Test, $p > .05$). Therefore, the differentiation in independent and dependent subjects seems not to be relevant for the valuation of the health states.

The EuroQol visual analogue scale as a school grade.

From discussions during the pilot study, the impression was gained that subjects saw the EuroQol visual analogue scale as a way to give a school grade or school mark to a health state. Thus, after finishing the questionnaire, the students were asked to give a mark to their own health state. In Holland, 10 is the best school grade, 0 the worst and 6 is sufficient to pass. The mean value of this mark was 8.152, with a standard deviation of 1.007. This value has a close resemblance to the value given on the visual analogue scale. On this scale, the students gave a mean value of 81.25 to their own health state, with a standard deviation of 10.22. The correlation between these 2 values was .7511. If it is true that people see the values on the EuroQol Instrument as school grades, then a value of 100 does not mean sufficient but excellent and 60 means sufficient.

The treatment of dead and unconscious.

The valuation of death has always been a point of discussion within the EuroQol Group and much research has been done on this topic. There is some evidence that the inclusion of the valuation of death may decrease the response, because it causes cognitive and emotional stress (see for instance EuroQolus topic 10). The mean value of death on the EuroQol visual analogue scale is always above 0 and has a high variance. Even values of 100 are reported (Brooks, 1991). The valuation of death also has theoretical complications (EuroQolus 10; van Hout, Rotterdam 7:11). The difficulty of valuing death was also visible in the results of this investigation. When asked what they would have done if the box labelled 'unconscious' had been labelled 'death', the students gave heterogeneous responses. These responses are listed in Table 7.5.

Table 7.5 Responses to the valuation of death on the EuroQol visual analog scale

Response	N	%
0	51	48.6
A value between 1 and 50	21	20.0
Death is not a health state (no value given)	26	24.7
A value between 50 and 1.00	3	2.9
"You can't be dead for 1 year'	2	1.9
A value below 0	1	1.0
'Don't know'	1	1.0
Total	105	100

As can be seen in Table 7.5, most subjects gave the value 0 or said that it was impossible to value death. About one quarter of the students gave a value between 0 and 100, which lifted the mean value of death above the theoretical anchor point of 0. Three students did not give a value to the state unconscious, because they felt it was not possible to do so. Many other students made spontaneous remarks or had to giggle when they valued unconscious and death. There was no doubt that the valuation of death and unconscious was a bizarre thing to do in their eyes.

The estimated time to complete the questionnaire.

It took an average of 12.85 minutes to complete the whole questionnaire and 6.92 minutes to value the health states. This last period of time did not include the reading of the instructions. At the end of the questionnaire the subjects were asked to estimate the time spent. The average estimated time was 13.42 minutes. The correlation between these two values was .568.

We concluded that the EuroQol Instrument was more easily administered compared to Standard Gamble (SG) and Time-Trade-Off (TTO). The EuroQol Instrument seems a simple way to elicit valuations for health states: these findings support its use for postal surveys.

Presented at the EuroQol Plenary Meeting: Helsinki, Finland, 1992

7.4 REFERENCES

Ashby J, O'Hanlon J, Rushby J. Health Questionnaire, Results of pilot testing. Internal note of the EuroQol Group 20/9/1988, ECOG, 1988.

Björk S, editor. EuroQol Conference Proceedings. Lund, October 1991. Discussion Paper No 1. In: IHE Working paper 1992:2. Lund, 1992.

Brooks R G, Jendteg S, Lindgren B, Persson U, Björk S. EuroQol: health-related quality of life measurement. Results of the Swedish questionnaire exercise. Health Policy 1991;18:37-48.

Carr-Hill R A. A second opinion: Health related quality of life measurement - Euro Style. Health Policy 1992;20:321-328.

Essink-Bot M L, Bonsel G J, Maas P J van der. Valuation of health states by the general public: feasibility of a standardized measurement procedure. Soc. Sci. Med. Vol. 1990;31(11):1201-1206.

EuroQol Group. EuroQol - A new facility for the measurement of health-related quality of life. Health Policy 1990;16:199-208.

EuroQol Group. Not a quick fix. Health Service Journal 21/11/1991, 1991.

EuroQol Group. EuroQol - A reply and reminder. Health Policy, 1992;20:329-328.

Nord E. EuroQol: health-related quality of life measurement. Valuations of health states by the general public in Norway. Health Policy 1991;18:25-36.

Nord E. A list of EuroQol papers and a systematic list of EuroQol points (the 'Index EuroQolus"). Internal note of the EuroQol Group 14/3/1991, 1991.

Sutherland H J, Llewellyn-Thomas H, Boyd N F, Till J E. Attitude toward quality of survival: The concept of maximal endurable time. Medical Decision Making 1982;2(3):229-309.

8
Eliciting EuroQol descriptive data and utility scale values from inpatients

Caroline Selai and Rachel Rosser

8.1 SUMMARY

We conducted a microstudy to elicit health state descriptions and utility values, using the EuroQol Instrument, from a sample of acutely ill inpatients on 5 wards at University College London Medical School. Most current work to date has elicited such descriptive and valuation data from random surveys of the general population. One problem with this is that most responders from the general population have not actually experienced the states being valued. Our goal was to ascertain whether there were any differences between the values given by inpatients and those of the general population. However, the small sample size of patients included in our feasibility study means our conclusions must remain tentative. Nevertheless the results suggest that patients give higher values than the general population. We suggest that more research needs to be done eliciting values from patients.

The measurement of patients' health-related quality of life is acknowledged to be important for a number of reasons, including the assessment of outcome of healthcare interventions. In a climate of economic scarcity, decisions about the allocation of healthcare resources need to be made explicit. The EuroQol Instrument has been devised to collect both qualitative quality-of-life (QoL) data and explicit valuations of health states.

The EuroQol Instrument aims to fulfil a specific and important role in HRQoL evaluation, and one that had not previously been attempted. It was conceived at a time when there was an exponential increase in the number of HRQoL measures being developed for various uses. With HRQoL data being elicited by such diverse methods for different goals, systematic evaluation and comparison of the data and of the methodologies used was difficult and often impossible.

This issue was the main focus of a group of QoL researchers from centres in 5 northern European countries who first met in 1987 to pool their multidisciplinary expertise and experience. The Group agreed that some mechanism was required to assist comparison of data between studies and between nations; that is, a linkage tool using a basic common core of HRQoL criteria. Consequently, the EuroQol Instrument was designed to describe the basic minimum elements of HRQoL. It was envisaged that it would be used alongside other instruments that were considered appropriate to the

P. Kind et al. (eds.), EQ-5D concepts and methods, 91–107.

particular study design. The EuroQol Instrument was designed to have the properties of both a single index and a health profile.

To fulfil the properties of the single index, a composite-state scaling task was devised that incorporated the state of 'being dead', which facilitated the construction of a cardinal index scale from zero (dead) to 1 (health). This does not rule out the existence of states considered worse than death. Thus, data elicited using the EuroQol Instrument can inform economic calculations such as the quality-adjusted life year (QALY).

The background to and aims of the EuroQol Group, the development of the EuroQol questionnaire and the results of a preliminary cross-national data analysis are outlined in the EuroQol Group's first publication (EuroQol Group, 1990). A second EuroQol Group publication giving an update of the current status of EuroQol research is currently in preparation.

It is important to be mindful that the EuroQol Instrument, which is designed to be a linkage tool, has certain constraints, and to remember that the questionnaire will not meet any QoL researcher's every need.

Since that first paper (EuroQol Group, 1990), the EuroQol descriptive classification has been modified and subsequently frozen for a period to allow lessons to be learned about the psychometric properties of the instrument. Version 2 of the EuroQol descriptive system is shown in Table 8.1.

Table 8.1 The EuroQol descriptive system (version 2)

Dimension	Level	Level description
Mobility	1	No problems walking about
	2	Some problems walking about
	3	Confined to bed
Self-care	1	No problems with self-care
	2	Some problems washing or dressing self
	3	Unable to wash or dress self
Usual activities	1	No problems with performing usual activities (e.g. work, study, housework, family and leisure activities)
	2	Some problems performing usual activities
	3	Unable to perform usual activities
Pain/discomfort	1	No pain or discomfort
	2	Moderate pain or discomfort
	3	Extreme pain or discomfort
Anxiety/depression	1	Not anxious or depressed
	2	Moderately anxious or depressed
	3	Extremely anxious or depressed

This is the latest version of the EuroQol Instrument and has been operational since 1991. The EuroQol Instrument is used to describe an individual's health state in terms of a 5-digit code number, each digit of which relates to the corresponding level of each dimension. The dimensions are always listed in the order given in Table 8.1; thus, the health state '11232' means:

- no problems in walking about (1)
- no problems with self-care (1)
- some problems with performing usual activities (2)
- extreme pain or discomfort (3)
- moderately anxious or depressed (2).

There are 2 more health states that lie outside this classification, those of unconscious and death. Thus, the EuroQol Instrument describes 245 theoretically possible health states.

Reliability and validity testing of the EuroQol Instrument are ongoing. Work is also being undertaken to use the EuroQol Instrument alongside other HRQoL measures such as the Short-Form 36 Health Survey (SF-36), the General Health Questionnaire (GHQ) and the Nottingham Health Profile (NHP). In addition, the valuing of the state 'being dead' has highlighted considerable methodological complexities, and this is the subject of further research being conducted by part of the EuroQol Group. The EuroQol Instrument has been translated into several languages, and is currently being used worldwide (Nord, 1991; Sintonen, 1993).

Within the field of HRQoL research there is ongoing discussion concerning various technical issues, both specific to the EuroQol questionnaire (Carr-Hill, 1992; EuroQol Group, 1992) and pertaining to HRQoL measures in general (Rosser, 1990; Selai and Rosser, 1993). One of these is the question of whose utility values should be obtained. This subsumes issues such as whether it is most appropriate to ask a representative sample of the population and, if so, what is the appropriate sampling frame? In a hypothetical scaling exercise, can volunteers from the general population value and compare health states of which they have no direct experience? Given that scaling tasks (exercises in which respondents are asked to assign numerical values to different health states) yield a broad range of values, should we aggregate these data and take the mean or median figure? What should we do if values in one geographical area differ from those in another?

Different groups of individuals do give different utility values. In addition, the values of individuals change throughout their lifetime; for example, the attitude of an older, married person with good family support towards disfigurement may differ from that of an adolescent. Also, societal values and attitudes to health, diet, economic roles and gender stereotyping are constantly changing, with attendant psychosocial sequelae for the individual. There is some evidence to suggest that sociodemographic variables affect utility valuations (Sackett and Torrance, 1978; Froberg and Kane, 1978). Studies have shown that differences in valuations also depend on experience of illness and level of neuroticism (Rosser and Kind, 1978).

However, from the existing literature, we do not have a clear picture as to which interpersonal variables influence utility values. It is against this background that we undertook a preliminary study to collect both descriptive and scaling data from inpatients at a teaching hospital in London, England. In other words, patients were asked both to describe their current health state and to complete the EuroQol health valuation task. Much work has looked at how patients rate their quality of life (Walker and Rosser, 1978; Fallowfield, 1990). Results have varied, and have included the finding that severely mobility-impaired people assess their quality of life as being quite high (Stensman, 1985). Although less work has been done with inpatients completing scaling exercises, there is evidence to suggest that valuations made by patients and healthy volunteers are different (Sackett and Torrance, 1978). Rosser and Kind (Rosser and Kind, 1978) conducted interviews in 70 individuals, including medical and psychiatric patients, and found differences in scale values between the various groups taking part. Significant differences between the values of doctors, medical patients and medical nurses were found.

There was closest agreement between psychiatric patients and their nurses, and between medical patients and their nurses (Rosser and Kind, 1978). The study presented here is, to our knowledge, the first attempt to elicit EuroQol scaling values from a sample of inpatients. The EuroQol Group is currently working to elicit values for all of the health states in the EuroQol Instrument [mainly from members of the general population of each of the member countries (Denmark, Finland, Norway, The Netherlands, Spain, Sweden and the UK)]. We undertook this pilot study for 2 reasons:

(i) the *a priori* desirability of asking patients to give values; and
(ii) the need to conduct a pilot study to ascertain the feasibility of eliciting these data from inpatients.

The aims of the study were:

(i) to elicit and compare self-reported ratings of health-related quality of life in a sample of acutely ill people;
(ii) to obtain their scaling values using 2 techniques (the 3-D Rosser Index Scaling Task (Rosser, 1993a) and the EuroQol Instrument); and
(iii) to compare EuroQol health state values obtained from inpatients with those obtained from the general population.

8.2 METHODS

We performed a micro-study of acutely ill inpatients in a busy London teaching hospital [University College London Medical School (UCLMS), London, England].

The results of the 3-D Rosser Index Scaling Task are currently in preparation. By pooling these data with data already collected by the EuroQol Group, comparisons may be made between the EuroQol health state values obtained from inpatients and those obtained from the general population.

Permission to interview patients was obtained from consultants (and their multidisciplinary care teams) on 5 wards at the UCLMS. Patients on 2 surgical (general surgery and orthopaedics) and 3 medical (neurology, oncology and adolescent oncology) wards were studied.

The field investigator (C.S.) visited the wards periodically over a 3-month period. Nursing staff were consulted to ascertain which patients were too ill to be approached. The nursing staff on the 5 wards were contacted at the beginning of each week and arrangements were made for the field researcher to visit the ward at an appropriate time, subject to the timetabling of doctors' ward rounds, etc. Patients were selected by nursing staff if they were well enough to be approached. Patients who could potentially be included were randomly selected; that is, there were no inclusion/exclusion criteria. However, no patient was approached without prior consultation with nursing staff concerning the patient's ability and willingness to be interviewed. The field researcher was introduced to the patients by the nurse. Ethical approval for the project having been granted by the UCLMS Ethics Committee, informed consent was obtained from each patient before proceeding with the interview.

The questionnaires were shown to the patients, and it was briefly explained that valuing health states was important for a number of reasons such as comparing the benefits of different health treatments. Patients were offered both instruments; the 3-D Rosser Index Scaling Task was always offered first, the EuroQol second. Both questionnaires are self-completed, but the researcher stayed at the bedside to answer any queries.

The full EuroQol Instrument was administered as follows:

(i) the patient described their current health state;
(ii) the patient rated their current health state on a visual analogue scale from zero to 100; and
(iii) the patient valued the composite health states, also on a zero to 100 visual analogue scale.

8.3 RESULTS

In total, 48 inpatients were approached during the 3-month study period. Of these 48, 8 patients (17%) refused to be interviewed. One of these patients refused because they were awaiting the arrival of a clinician to perform a test. The other 7 refused because they felt too ill to undergo an interview. All 40 patients who consented to be interviewed completed the 3-D Rosser Index Scaling Task. The results of these interviews are not presented here. Of these 40 patients, 23 (58%) went on to complete the EuroQol. The 17 patients who completed the 3-D Rosser Index Scaling Task but not the EuroQol left the study at that point for a number of reasons. First, the high patient turnover at UCLMS meant that 5 patients who had agreed to be interviewed, and whose second interviews were postponed until the completion of a clinical procedure, were not seen before they were discharged. Some patients (n = 11) stated that they could not go on to the second scaling exercise because of fatigue. One patient withdrew after the 3-D Rosser Index Scaling Task because of Parkinson's disease, which created difficulties in completing the interviews.

For patients who completed both the 3-D Rosser Index and the EuroQol scaling tasks, the total interview time ranged from 20 to 60 minutes (mean 42 minutes). The time spent on the EuroQol ranged from 5 to 30 minutes (mean 18 minutes).

Table 8.2 shows the age, gender and diagnosis of participants as reported by the patients themselves. The results of the EuroQol Instrument study are shown in Table 8.3. Table 8.3 also shows the mean scores for each health state. The mean of the mean scores for all health states was 51.1.

Individuals completing the EuroQol scaling task were asked to rate 'being dead' on 2 separate pages of the questionnaire. This was done to allow some assessment of the consistency and stability of respondents' answers. Table 8.4 shows the values given for the state 'being dead' elicited from the inpatient sample.

The inpatients had few problems in establishing their own health state (by ticking the boxes of the self-rated descriptive classification) or in rating their own health on the visual analogue scale. Some patients made comments about both the EuroQol and 3-D Rosser Index Scaling Tasks, most of which were requests for clarification. However, the respondents had some problems in comprehending the task and understanding its relevance.

Interestingly, respondents had considerably more comments about the specific task of rating 'being dead' than for the other health states. These comments were broadly philosophical in nature and are too lengthy to include here. Interested readers should write to the authors for details. On the whole, patients were not apparently distressed by this task, but their comments and the results (Table 8.4) show that they had many difficulties in making such a judgement. Several of the patients rated 'being dead' as having quite a high utility and even, in some cases, as being the 'best possible' health state (score = 100). One of these patients had been admitted for a knee replacement operation, and the other had leg ulceration. However, one patient, who was on an orthopaedic ward, complained to the nursing staff that this question had upset him, and the research had to be suspended temporarily pending clarification of the task and its potential to upset patients in general.

Table 8.2 Demographic characteristics of the patients as reported by themselves

Patient no.	Gender	Age (years)	Ward specialty	Diagnosis as reported by patient[a]	3-D	EuroQol
1	F	43	Orth	Hip replacement	✓	✓
2	M	33	GS	Leg thrombosis	✓	✓
3	M	75	Orth	Replacement knee operation	✓	×
4	M	36	Orth	Foot infection secondary to road traffic accident	✓	✓
5	M	68	GS	Blocked coronary artery (bypass operation)	✓	✓
6	F	49	CS	Rectal pain (sigmoidoscopy)	✓	✓
7	F	20	GS	Appendix/ovaries (scan)	✓	×
8	F	58	CS	Venous ulcer	✓	✓
9	F	60	Orth	Rheumatoid arthritis	✓	✓
10	M	39	N[b]	Severe atopic eczema	✓	✓
11	F	71	Orth	Knee replacement operation	✓	✓
12	F	65	GS	Leg amputation	✓	×
13	F	28	N	For neurological investigations	✓	✓
14	F	24	N	Leg ulcers	✓	✓
15	F	27	GS	Axillary cyst removal	✓	✓
16	M	60	N	Parkinson's disease	✓	×
17	M	65	N	Parkinson's disease	✓	×
8	F	27	N	Epilepsy and pregnancy	✓	✓
19	F	40	CS	Varicose veins	✓	×
20	M	59	GS	'Leg blockages'	✓	×
21	M	52	CS	Hernia repair	✓	×
22	F	42	Onc	Lymphoma	✓	✓
23	F	52	Onc	Granulocytic sarcoma	✓	✓
24	M	72	Onc	Stomach cancer	✓	×
25	M	51	Onc	Oesophageal cancer	✓	✓
26	M	44	Onc	Cancer	✓	✓
27	F	48	Onc	Cancer	✓	×
28	F	46	CS	Sciatica	✓	×
29	M	30	Onc	Terminal lung cancer	✓	×
30	M	54	CS	'Lower leg blockage'	✓	×
31	F	64	GS	Leg blockage (bypass operation)	✓	×
32	M	33	Onc	Rhabdomyosarcoma	✓	✓
33	F	29	N	Weakness and pain	✓	✓
34	M	56	N	Parkinson's disease	✓	×
35	M	52	Onc	Lung cancer	✓	✓
36	F	29	AO	Cancer	✓	✓
37	F	20	AO	Bone tumour	✓	✓
38	M	58	CS	Arterial blockage in leg	✓	×
39	F	16	AO	Acute lymphoblastic leukaemia	✓	✓
40	M	59	N	Parkinson's disease	✓	×

a Patients' stated reason for hospitalisation is given because patients' appraisal of their quality of life depends on what they believe to be their current problem.

b Overflow from dermatology ward.

Abbreviations: 3-D = 3-D Rosser Index Scaling Task; AO) = adolescent oncology; F = female; GS = general surgery; M = male; N = neurology; Onc = oncology; Orth = orthopaedic surgery.

Table 8.3 Results of the EuroQol scaling task. For an explanation of health state notation, see Introduction and Table 8.1. The numbers in the table represent the patient's self-rating of numerous hypothetical health states on a visual analogue scale from zero to 100. Patients were asked to value health states 11111 and 33333 twice to assess consistency and stability

		Health state being valued																
Patient no.	Health state[a]	own health state	11211	11111	21232	11122	11121	22233	33333	33321	21111	11111	Unc.	12111	11112	32211	33333	22323
1	22231	30	86	90	30	40	92	45	85	45	80	90	27	65	86	60	65	55
2	11122	90	70	75	75	75	75	50	30	35	60	86	50	60	70	40	10	30
3	32312	30	100	60	70	20	10	50	85	100	50	80	60	67	10	25		
4	21232	42	80	30	20	30	50	40	20	20	20	30	13	20	20	20	20	30
5	11111	90	90	90	60	40	60	30	0	10	90	98	100	70	80	10	0	20
6	22221	94	98	95	94	95	95	90	80	80	98	100	10	84	85	80	60	80
7	21211	80	98	90	60	75	75	50	30	40	92	93	60	80	90	80	30	50
8	11111	85	60	50	85	5	5											
9	21222	60	95	100	40	95	75	30	0	20	90	100	100	45	85	40	0	50
10	21222	60	95	100	70	60	100	30	8	30	50	100	0	90	90	30	10	30
11	11221	95	60	100	45	60	80	30	0	0	85	100	10	60	90	40	40	0
12	12222	70	60	66	70	56	60	60	86	57	85	72	70	70	84	70	54	55
13	11212	70	75	95	25	30	70	30	10	15	80	85	0	50	40	20	10	10
14[b]	21222	50																
15	21211	100	90	100	10	20	40	15	0	0	60	100	40	50	98	40	0	0
16	11122	45	90	70	30	40	70	70	30	20	90	90	40	40	90	30	10	0
17	1132[c]	30	75	100	50		85	50	20	35	85	100	10	50	75	65	40	30
18	21311	75	80	100	25	40	74	18	4	18	70	100	15	80	65	46	10	25
19	21321	35	90	90	30	50	70	30	0	20	80	100	5	60	70	30	0	30
20	22322	35	85	75	47	100	83	56	24	24	50		17	100	96	40	30	60
21	11222	80	90	100	30	50	90	30	0	20	90	100	13	30	85	20	7	
22	21322	45	73	80	30	40	50	15	40	25	65	84	30	40	40	35	5	20
23	11221	85	90	100	40	60	95	30	5	20	90	100	70	95	85	80	10	30
Mean score		64.2	83.5	86.6	44.3	57.2	74.2	39.0	22.1	26.8	76.0	91.4	34.8	62.8	75.4	44.9	20.7	30.3
(SD)		(24.0)	(11.5)	(17.9)	(21.1)	(23.0)	(16.0)	(19.1)	(27.8)	(19.1)	(19.0)	(16.4)	(30.8)	(21.7)	(2[illegible].4)	(21.7)	(20.9)	(21.6)

a Health state at the time of the interview.

b No valuation data are available because the patient did not understand the questionnaire.

c No rating available for anxiety/depression.

Abbreviations: SD = standard deviation; Unc. = unconscious.

Table 8.4 Valuations for the state 'being dead' in the EuroQol scaling task. Patients were asked to value this state (on a visual analogue scale from zero to 100) on 2 separate pages of the questionnaire, to allow assessment of consistency and stability

Patient no.	First valuation	Second valuation
1	0.6	0.6
2	5.0	5.0
3	5.0	5.0
4	0.0	0.0
5	0.0	0.0
6[a]		
7[a]		
8[a]		
9	100.0	100.0
10[b]		
11	100.0	100.0
12[b]		
13	0.0	0.0
14	6.4	3.4
15	0.0	0.0
16	0.6	a
17[a]		
18	0.4	0.5
19	1.0	1.0
20[a]		
21	0.0	0.0
22	4.0	4.0
23	7.5	7.5
Mean	14.4	15.1

a Patient did not attempt question.

b Patient wrote too difficult' or 'cannot answer'.

8.4 DISCUSSION

The results of the present study can be compared with those of 3 previously conducted health state valuation studies that also used the EuroQol Instrument (Table 8.5)(EuroQol Group, 1990). These studies were conducted in Lund (Sweden), Frome (England) and Bergen op Zoom (BoZ) [The Netherlands], and their results are discussed in the first corporate EuroQol paper (EuroQol Group, 1990). The respondents in these studies were a random sample of the general population. The results of the present study show a wide range of scores for each health state rated (Table 8.3); the large standard deviations obtained should alert us to the questionable validity of the mean scores. We calculated the overall mean of the mean values for both our data (see 8.3 Results) and that obtained in the 3 pilot studies (Table 8.5) (EuroQol Group, 1990). Although these data must be interpreted with caution, it is interesting to note that the mean of the means for the inpatient group is much higher than that of any of the 3 published groups (51.1 vs 39, 39 and 41, respectively). This suggests that the patients valued the health states as having a higher utility than the general population. In an earlier study conducted by Rosser and Kind (Rosser and Kind, 1978), psychiatric patients gave the highest valuations out of all those studied. The medically ill patients gave relatively low figures (Rosser and Kind, 1978). However, it is difficult to compare this earlier study (Rosser and Kind, 1978) with the present one because of the differences in study population (psychiatric and medical patients). In the original study (Rosser and Kind, 1978), one patient became very distressed after a rejected transplanted kidney was removed, necessitating the patient's return to dialysis. This patient had been in every one of the 29 health states studied by Rosser and Kind (Rosser and Kind, 1978) in the previous month.

As shown in Table 8.4, 2 inpatients rated the state of 'being dead' as having very high utility. The phenomenon of rating this state as the best possible health state is not unknown to the EuroQol Group, and some members have previously carried out research on this topic (Kind and Rosser, 1979). This issue has prompted the formation of a special 'working party' EuroQol subgroup to look specifically at the issues surrounding the valuation of 'being dead'. However, one important lesson to be learned from this study is that the result of one patient being upset by the question had far-reaching consequences (the temporary suspension of research on that ward). The ratings for the state 'being dead' (Table 8.4) show that the patients had great difficulty in attempting this task. This finding, plus the fact that some patients had complained to their nursing staff that rating 'being dead' had upset them, leads us to the conclusion that this question cannot be asked of some seriously ill patients without empathic and tentative discussion. In some instances, the question should perhaps be omitted from the discussion.

We could explore the question differently and ask the patient what they would choose if they were given a choice, and why they made that choice. There is a difference between choosing (preferring) the state 'being dead' and the actual condition of 'being dead'. Death might be quite rationally chosen instead of the patient's least preferred health state. The issue of 'being dead' is pertinent to the current euthanasia debate, which is outside the scope of this article.

The mean utility values given by inpatients for the state 'being dead' (Table 8.4) can be compared with the previously published means in Table 8.5. The means of the inpatients' values (15.1 and 14.4) are rather higher than the data obtained in the Lund (10 and 10) and Frome (10 and 10) studies (Table 8.5) and are nearer to the means obtained in the BoZ study (19 and 18). These differences suggest that more research needs to be done with a much larger sample to ascertain whether patients systematically value health states differently from the general population. The issue of which 'tariff' of health states to choose is at the centre of philosophical debates about the context in which such data should be used.

Table 8.5 Results of 3 pilot studies conducted with the EuroQol Instrument in 3 centres: (i) Lund, Sweden; (ii) Frome, England; and (iii) Bergen op Zoom, The Netherlands (BoZ) (EuroQol Group, 1990, with permission). For an explanation of health state notation, see 8.1 Summary and Table 8.1. The data in the table are the mean valuations given by participants for each health state, ranging from zero (worst) to 100 (best)

	Mean valuations (SD)		
Health state[a,b]	Lund	Frome	BoZ
111111	93(13)	95(10)	93(13)
111121	83(16)	81(14)	81(19)
111112	69(21)	67(18)	71(22)
111122	64(20)	65(17)	69(21)
112121	61(22)	67(18)	63(23)
112131	51(21)	56(19)	56(22)
112222[a]	36(20)	41(17)	43(21)
112222[c]	38(19)	40(16)	41(21)
112232	36(20)	36(17)	37(23)
212232	26(20)	26(16)	26(20)
222232	14(19)	12(12)	12(15)
232232	12(19)	8(9)	10(16)
322232	9(18)	5(7)	10(18)
332232	8(19)	4(6)	7(12)
Being dead[a]	10(24)	10(20)	19(25)
Being dead[c]	10(23)	10(21)	18(25)
Mean of mean values	39	39	41

a First valuation.

b Each health state has 6 digits because the original descriptive classification had 6 dimensions. The sixth dimension ('social') has now been incorporated into the 'usual activities' dimension.

c Second valuation.

Abbreviation: SD = standard deviation.

Since this was a feasibility study conducted in very small numbers of patients, the data are presented merely as an addition to the current EuroQol data pool. The conclusions we can draw from comparing Tables 8.3 and 8.5 are limited because the EuroQol questionnaire was modified between the Lund/Frome/BoZ data and the current data. At this stage, we were mainly concerned with the feasibility of eliciting health state valuations and values for the state 'being dead' from inpatients.

In the present study, in most cases, the patients' HRQoL self-ratings were surprisingly high (Table 8.3). For example, patient number 23 in Table 8.2, who had a diagnosis of granulocytic sarcoma, gave a selfrating of 21211, indicating that her health was apparently fine apart from some problems in walking about and in performing usual activities. These findings may be a function of the measurement technique or interviewing style. In the original valuation research (Rosser and Kind, 1978), the non-medical interviewer (there were 2 interviewers, one of whom was a psychiatrist) always obtained the middle figures. This may be explained by complex issues such as patient fear or apprehension resulting in denial or cognitive dissonance (i.e. patients may deny that they are as ill as they actually are), guilt about being in hospital or anxiety that they might be discharged prematurely.

It is important to note that all that is asked for on the EuroQol is a description of the patient's health state on that day. Prognosis is not covered, but a profile can be built up by examining the description on subsequent days. Prognosis and the incidence profile (an incidence profile is the changing pattern of health state on any given day) are different things, both of which need to be taken into account when monitoring patients' quality of life over time. It has been argued that, for most current QoL instruments, time and time-related issues are in need of further research (Rosser, 1993b).

QoL researchers are engaged in ongoing debates concerning methodology and epistemology. There are many as yet unresolved issues pertaining to the best method for the elicitation of utility values, cross-cultural research methodology, the aggregation of data, the computation of a global index QoL score, and the use to which such summary data is put. Most of these issues are outside the scope of this article. However, this current research has been prompted by a specific concern about the elicitation of utility values: the idea of achieving consensus. Some of the issues pertaining to this are summarised as follows:

(a) The patients described their health state (boxes ticked in each of the domains) as 'fairly good'. A full discussion of this phenomenon, which can be explained in terms of patients' coping mechanisms or cognitive dissonance, is outside the scope of this article. However, it is an important issue (for all HRQoL instruments and not just the EuroQol) that has implications if indications of care and treatment are based on HRQoL scores. The under-reporting of seriously ill patients would have implications for the allocation of resources. Indeed, such findings reopen the debate about whether subjective or objective appraisals of quality of life are to be preferred.

(b) Should we strive to obtain views from patients as separate from the general population? What if their values are systematically different? Are they the best judges (because of their health/sickness experiences) or are they poor judges Although the HRQoL philosophy is a move away from the view that the expert knows best, allowing the patient to evaluate their own quality of life sometimes causes concern, such as when the patient has a low level of intellectual/cognitive functioning. However, use of surrogate informants is at present controversial. In a less clear-cut case, hospitalisation induces a further degree of anxiety in patients whose quality of life is already diminished by their condition.

It has been suggested that the views of patients before treatment are in some way invalid. For example, Morgado *et al,* (1991) asked patients to report the adequacy of several aspects of their lives before treatment with antidepressant medications. After treatment, they were asked to give ratings for the same period (i.e. before alleviation of the depression). Interestingly, patients gave statistically significantly lower scores (indicating a better quality of life) for that period. Hermann (1993), reviewing several such studies, stated that 'systematic biases can occur as a function of mood state and [have] the potential to affect assessment of quality of life'. The suggestion here is that there was a 'true' HRQoL description but that the patients, when depressed, were unable to perceive this correctly. Surely, however, if patients are depressed and perceive their quality of life to be poor, then the HRQoL score that they give is their 'true' HRQoL score at that time. Depression is debilitating and has a far-reaching impact on quality of life; the illness may not be a filter through which a patient 'incorrectly' judges the other aspects of their functioning.

In general, patients' evaluations are particularly important because they are experiencing symptoms (e.g. severe pain) and the psychosocial sequelae of their condition (e.g. stigma), which many of us have difficulty trying to imagine.

(c) For policy decision purposes, it has been suggested that researchers need to elicit the valuations of a very large number of people (2000 or more) from a variety of backgrounds (Williams, 1992). It is argued that in a world of scarcity and opportunity cost, choosing to treat one patient necessarily implies not treating some other person, and so the values of every affected or potentially affected person are surely relevant (Williams and Kind, 1992). However, there is concern that ratings provided by the general public may not reflect the values of patients in general, and in particular those of the patient(s) to be treated (Fallowfield, 1990; Spiegelhalter *et al,* 1992). Return rates from postal surveys are low (EuroQol Group, 1990) and there is clear systematic bias: replies will not be obtained from illiterate people, illegal immigrants, blind

people and frequent users of health services. More work needs to be done to explore the motivations of the responders.
If patients' values do systematically differ from those of the general population (and we suggest that further study is required in this area), then which set of values is to be used? This partly depends on the application of the data; the values obtained from different subsets of responders could be kept separate. However, users need to be aware of the origins of the tariff of values they use for their calculations.

The data reported in the present study are elementary. The large variance reported in all public surveys raises questions about the meaningfulness of the aggregated data. There is a shift in opinion away from direct elicitation of values from patients back to a mathematical modeling approach. However, it has yet to be shown whether preferences can be modelled and validated predictively.

8.5 CONCLUSIONS

The current issues surrounding the achievement of a single index score that reflects global quality of life pertain to both to the fundamental theories and to the practical issues. This article has not attempted to fully address the underlying assumptions concerning the elicitation of views from a representative sample of the population, the sampling frame, the aggregation of data and other issues. We have, however, raised 2 questions:

(i) whether patients' views should be incorporated into the overall data; and
(ii) whether such an exercise is feasible.

The answer to the first question remains an issue for debate. However, when considering the various uses of summary HRQoL scores, it becomes apparent that the answer to this question will have important political sequelae. The use of these data to inform decisions about the allocation of scarce resources raises important issues, such as the views of clinicians trying to respond to the wishes of their particular patients and to those of society, of which they are part. A clinician may experience a conflict between satisfying the needs of a particular patient and the overall needs of society.

In answer to the second question, we suggest that such an exercise is feasible. However, our experience has highlighted some of the problems of asking such a population to rate 'being dead'. Whether this limitation ultimately nullifies the value of eliciting utilities from patients altogether should be open to debate because, to reiterate, patients are experiencing what most of us attempting these scaling tasks can only imagine.

We set out to conduct a feasibility study on a small sample of acutely ill patients. The small sample size precludes extensive data analyses, and conclusions must be tentative. However, we conclude that it is feasible to elicit EuroQol self-ratings and utility values from acutely ill inpatients with the possible exception of eliciting a rating for the state 'being dead'.

More empirical work needs to be done in the field of eliciting evaluations from the seriously ill, and more theoretical work needs to be done to reappraise the aggregation of data and the appropriate measure of central tendency. These will both have implications for the use of summary QoL scores to inform economic decisions about healthcare.

8.6 ACKNOWLEDGEMENTS

We gratefully acknowledge: the assistance of the other members of the EuroQol Group; the Middlesex Hospital Clinical Investigations Panel for granting ethical consent for this research project; and consultants, colleagues and patients who agreed to take part in this study.

Presented at the EuroQol Plenary Meeting: Rotterdam, The Netherlands, 1993

8.7 REFERENCES

Carr-Hill R A. A second opinion: health related quality of life measurement - Euro style. Health Policy 1992;20:321-329.

EuroQol Group. EuroQol - a new facility for the measurement of health related quality of life. Health Policy 1990;16:199-208.

EuroQol Group. EuroQol - a reply and reminder. Health Policy 1992;20:329-32.

Fallowfield L. Quality of life: the missing measurement in health care. Human Horizons Series. London: Souvenir Press (E&A) Ltd., 1990.

Froberg D, Kane R. Methodology for measuring health preferences III: population and context effects. J Clin Epidemiol 1978;42:585-592.

Hermann B P. Developing a model of quality of life in epilepsy: the contribution of neuropsychology. Epilepsia 1993;34(4):14-21.

Kind P, Rosser R M. Death & dying: scaling of death for health status indices. In: Barber B, Gremy F, Uberla K, et al, editors. Lecture notes on medical informatics. Springer-Verlag, 1979:28-36.

Morgado A, Raoux N, Jourdain G, *et al.* Over-reporting of maladjustment by depressed subjects. Soc Psychiatry Psychiatr Epidemiol 1991;26:68-74.

Nord E. EuroQol: health-related quality of life measurement. Valuations of health states by the general public in Norway. Health Policy 1991;18:25-36.

Rosser R M, Kind P. A scale of valuations of states of illness: is there a social consensus? Int J Epidemiol 1978;7(4):347-358

Rosser R M. From health indicators to quality adjusted life years: technical and ethical issues. In: Hopkins A, Costain D, editors. Measuring the outcomes of medical care. London: RCP Publications, 1990:1-16.

Rosser R M. A health index and output measure. In: Walker S R, Rosser R M, editors. Quality of life assessment: key issues in the 1990s. London: Kluwer Academic Publishers, 1993a:151-178.

Rosser R M. Forwards to the past: some thorny issues revisited. Paper presented at a joint meeting of the WHO and Foundation Ipsen; 1993 Jul 2-3: Paris, 1993b.

Sackett D, Torrance G. The utility of different health states as perceived by the general public. J Chronic Dis 1978;31:697-704.

Selai C E, Rosser R M. Good quality quality? Some methodological issues. J R Soc Med 1993;86:440-443.

Sintonen H, editor. Discussion paper no. 2. EuroQol conference proceedings: Helsinki. Kuopio: Department of Social Sciences, University of Kuopio, 1993.

Spiegelhalter D J, Gore S M, Fitzpatrick R, *et al.* Quality of life measures in health care III: Resource allocation. BMJ 1992;305:1205-1209.

Stensman R. Severely mobility disabled people assess the quality of their lives. Scand J Rehabil Med 1985;17:87-99.

Walker S W, Rosser R M, editors. Quality of life assessment: key issues in the 1990s. London: Kluwer Academic Publishers, 1993.

Williams A W, Kind P. The present state of play about QALYs. In: Hopkins A, editor. Measures of the quality of life and the uses to which such measures may be put. London: RCP Publications, 1992:21-39.

Williams A W. The importance of quality of life in policy decision making. In: Walker S R, Rosser R M, editors. Quality of life assessment: key issues in the 1990s. London: Kluwer Academic Publishers, 1993:427-439.

9
Test-retest reliability of health state valuations collected with the EuroQol questionnaire

Heleen van Agt, Marie-Louise Essink-Bot, Paul Krabbe and Gouke Bonsel

9.1 ABSTRACT

This study is a contribution by the Dutch participants to the research programme of the EuroQol Group. This collaborative group of researchers engaged in outcome measurement is working towards the development of a standardized, non-disease-specific instrument for describing and particularly valuing health-related quality of life. The present article analyses the test-retest reliability of the valuations collected with the EuroQol questionnaire in a population survey (n = 208). The choice of the appropriate method for test-retest analysis is discussed and the results of several approaches with the EuroQol data are shown.

Generalizability Theory is proposed as the most suitable method. This method is the most comprehensive, giving distinct information about the relative contributions of different sources of variance. The EuroQol valuations appear to have good test-retest reliability.

Keywords:

Generalizability Theory, Estimated variance component, EuroQol, Health state valuations, Level of measurement, Reliability.

9.2 INTRODUCTION

Since 1987, the EuroQol Group has been developing a standard non-disease-specific instrument for describing and valuing HRQoL. The Group's ultimate goal is to provide those engaged in economic evaluation of health care with a measurement procedure that generates in a feasible way universal (general) descriptions of patients' health status, to which representative values or utilities may be assigned in a second stage. These valuations may be obtained from a sample of the general public, independent of data collection from patients. Our study is a contribution to the Group's systematic investigation of the psychometric and other methodological properties of such a two-stage measurement instrument for economic valuation of health status. The following considerations have been taken into account in the design of the EuroQol measurement procedure (for details see Rosser and Sintonen, 1993). First, a descriptive classification was chosen consisting of five non-disease-specific dimen-

P. Kind et al. (eds.), EQ-5D concepts and methods, 109–123.

sions, similar to those in conventional generic health measures such as SIP (Bergner *et al*, 1976) and NHP (Hunt *et al*, 1986). Next, the EuroQol Group developed a valuation procedure which assigns a numerical value to each health state described by means of this classification. This valuation task applies visual analogue scaling (VAS) to a composite health state description referring as much as possible to a real-life patient's situation. In a technical sense we regard the continuum of values for all health states presented, defined by the end-points of the scale, as a quantitative reflection of the internal representation of the trait "valuation of health status". Since feasibility of the whole procedure was a major criterion during all the developmental work, the descriptive system is not too complex and the valuation task was designed to be suitable for unsupported large-scale data collection (postal surveys).

The current version of the EuroQol measurement procedure apparently provides a logical ranking of health states. Moreover respondents produce highly consistent answer patterns at the individual and the group levels. A striking similarity of the valuations obtained in different European countries was demonstrated (Essink-Bot *et al*, 1990; EuroQol Group, 1990; Nord, 1991; Brooks *et al*, 1991; EuroQol Group, 1992a). Sensitivity for non-response bias and for variations in socioeconomic background variables appeared to be low (EuroQol Group, 1992b; Essink-Bot et al, 1993).

The issue for this paper is the determination of test-retest reliability of the valuations. Reliability refers to the accuracy of a measurement instrument and is commonly operationalized as reproducibility of results. Test-retest reliability refers to the ability of a measurement instrument to produce the same results on two or more occasions, while it is assumed that the characteristic under study has remained unchanged. This is an important quality of a measurement instrument that is intended to measure a stable characteristic or 'trait'. In our case, it would be difficult to defend the use of health state valuations in health care allocation decisions if these valuations, as measured by the EuroQol questionnaire, where to change over time.

Specific attention is given to the method of analysing test-retest reliability since results usually depend on the method chosen. The Generalizability Theory (G-theory) was used for test-retest analysis because it appeared to be the most suitable method.
The study on test-retest reliability was part of a large population survey, the Rotterdam Survey as described in (EuroQol Group, 1992b; Essink-Bot et al, 1993).

9.3 MATERIAL AND METHODS

The EuroOol valuation questionnaire

The EuroQol concept of health consists of five dimensions, viz. Mobility, Self-care, Usual activities, Pain/Discomfort and Anxiety/Depression. Each dimension has three categories of the general form 'no problems' (level 1), 'some problems' (level 2), 'inability / extreme problems' (level 3). Health state descriptions can be composed by taking one level for each dimension. For example, state '11223' indicates a state of health without mobility or self-care problems, some problems with usual activities, moderate pain or discomfort, and extreme anxiety or depression. Theoretically 3^5 (243) composite health state descriptions are possible.

In the EuroQol valuation questionnaire, respondents are asked to value 16 health state descriptions 'for a person like yourself' on a visual analogue scale with marked end-points: 0 = 'worst imaginable health state' and 100 = 'best imaginable health state'. The duration of each state is supposed to be one year; what is going to happen afterwards is explicitly stated not to be known. One page of the questionnaire is shown in Figure 9.1.

The 16 health state descriptions are presented on two pages A and B. The standard EuroQol questionnaire contains a fixed selection of 14 different health states, while '11111' and '33333' are presented on both valuation pages of the questionnaire. In the Rotterdam Survey 14 additional health states were selected to be valued. Two new valuation pages were created (C, D). Four versions of the questionnaire were constructed, namely AB (standard EuroQol), CB, AD and CD. All health states occurred in two versions of the questionnaire, except '11111' and '33333', which occurred twice in each version.

As an introduction to the valuation task, respondents are requested to classify and rate their own state of health. Data on background characteristics are collected on the last page of the questionnaire.

The sample

The Rotterdam Survey was conducted with the EuroQol valuation questionnaire as a postal survey in a sample of 1400 households in Rotterdam, The Netherlands, in January 1991. Non-blank response amounted to 869 questionnaires (62%). For further details of the Rotterdam Survey, see (EuroQol Group, 1992b; Essink-Bot et al, 1993).

Respondents who had returned a non-blank questionnaire were asked if they were willing to participate in surveys of the same kind in the future. The 398 respondents who consented received a second questionnaire ('retest') in November 1991, consisting of, *inter alia,* the EuroQol valuation questionnaire. A reminder was sent two weeks later.

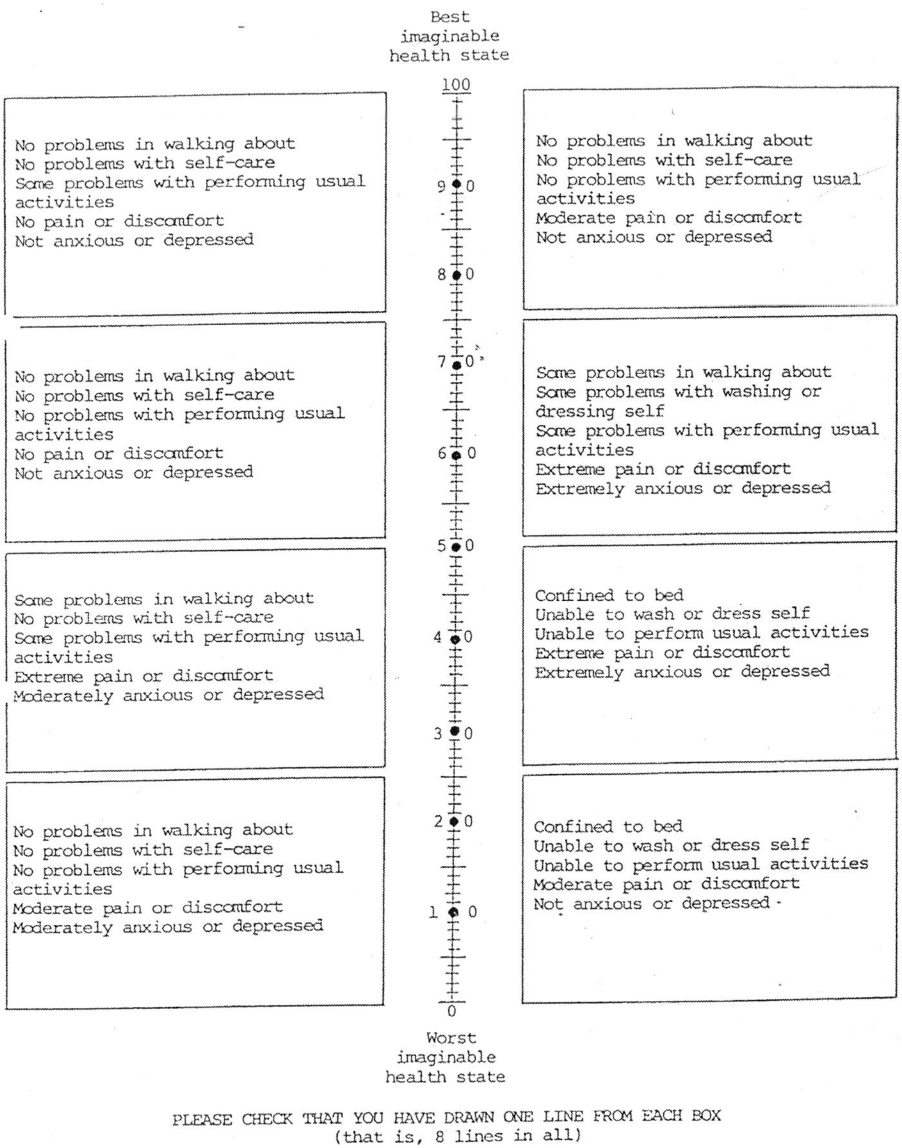
Best imaginable health state

100

No problems in walking about
No problems with self-care
Some problems with performing usual activities
No pain or discomfort
Not anxious or depressed

No problems in walking about
No problems with self-care
No problems with performing usual activities
Moderate pain or discomfort
Not anxious or depressed

90

80

No problems in walking about
No problems with self-care
No problems with performing usual activities
No pain or discomfort
Not anxious or depressed

Some problems in walking about
Some problems with washing or dressing self
Some problems with performing usual activities
Extreme pain or discomfort
Extremely anxious or depressed

70

60

50

Some problems in walking about
No problems with self-care
Some problems with performing usual activities
Extreme pain or discomfort
Moderately anxious or depressed

Confined to bed
Unable to wash or dress self
Unable to perform usual activities
Extreme pain or discomfort
Extremely anxious or depressed

40

30

No problems in walking about
No problems with self-care
No problems with performing usual activities
Moderate pain or discomfort
Moderately anxious or depressed

Confined to bed
Unable to wash or dress self
Unable to perform usual activities
Moderate pain or discomfort
Not anxious or depressed

20

10

0

Worst imaginable health state

PLEASE CHECK THAT YOU HAVE DRAWN ONE LINE FROM EACH BOX
(that is, 8 lines in all)

Figure 9.1 Page of the questionnaire

Statistics

Data were considered usable if at most 2 valuations were missing. If more valuations were missing, all data from this respondent were excluded. For 1 or 2 missing values, the median score of the rest of the population was filled in.

Data from individual respondents were defined as inconsistent if state 33333 was valued higher than or equal to state 11111 on one of the two valuation pages. In these cases all valuations from such a respondent were omitted from further analysis.

Background characteristics of all respondents in the test survey were compared with those of the respondents in the retest survey in order to recognize response selectivity.

Three determinants were identified for the choice of the appropriate method for analysis of the test-retest data (see also Table 9.1):

(i) The nature of the scores: analysis assuming interval measurement level or ordinal measurement level;
(ii) The level of stimulus aggregation: analysis per separate health state, or all health states simultaneously;
(iii) The level of respondent aggregation: analysis at the individual level, or at group level;

Table 9.1 Scheme for analysing test-retest reliability of health state valuations

	Interval		Ranks	
	per state	all states	per state	all states
individual	[irrelevant]	Pearson's correlaton	[irrelevant]	Kendall's W
group	ANOVA: Classical Test Theory	ANOVA: Generalizability Theory	ANOVA: Friedman by ranks	Kendall's W

(i)

Whether the use of valuations for constructing the valuation scale is justified, or whether the rank orderings of health states have to be used depends on the nature of the valuation scores. We used the multi-dimensional unfolding technique (MDU) by applying the ALSCAL model, to investigate whether the valuation scores could be regarded as interval or as ordinal data (Torgerson, 1958; Goombs, 1950; Takane *et al*, 1977). Unfolding theory assumes that the observed valuations are accounted for by one or more underlying dimensions. MDU derives the metric properties of the underlying scale of the health status continuum, here the relative distances between health states, by using information about the ordering of valuations of the individual respondents. The more sets of orderings of valuations are available, the more information can be derived about the metric properties of the underlying scale. We applied MDU by assuming one single underlying continuum to represent the health state valuation scale, considering first the valuations as ordinal data, then as interval data. If MDU assuming ordinal data provides similar results compared to MDU assuming interval data then the assumption that the valuations are interval data is justified. Conventional test-retest statistics usually require interval data by means of the Pearson correlation coefficient or a reliability coefficient (intra-class correlation) based on analysis of variance (ANOVA) (Streiner and Norman, 1989).

(ii)

The appropriate method depends also on the preferential level of stimulus aggregation. Deriving intra-class correlations on test-retest data from the EuroQol questionnaire would result in one coefficient per separate health state, allowing for only one source of variance (in this case: two moments of measurement) to be accounted for. The method of calculating the Pearson correlation coefficient allows us to analyse all health states simultaneously, resulting in one coefficient when applied at the group level. These methods do not give information about individual variation, unsell the Pearson correlation coefficients are derived for each respondent separately.

(iii)

From the economic viewpoint, however, we are primarily interested in the continuum of valuations of health states as rated by society. Therefore we focused on the aggregation of individual valuations to group level, assuming this would reflect the valuations of the population under study.

The appropriate approach should therefore analyze the effect of the moment of measurement, considering all health states and respondents simultaneously. In statistical terms we then need information about the relative contribution of specified sources of variation to the total amount of variation in the valuation data. The three specified sources of variation in our study are: the 16 health states, the 208 individual respondents, and the 2 moments of measurement. Only Generalizability Theory (GT) seems a suitable statistical technique for this approach, assuming interval metric properties of data (Streiner and Norman, 1989). Kendall's W coefficient of concordance, though an appropriate method to analyze rank data, is unable to show the relative contributions of different sources of variance (Siegel and Castellan, 1988). GT will be explained in more detail in the next section. The results of application of the other, partial, methods in Table 9.1 to this dataset have been published elsewhere (EuroQol Group, 1993).

Generalizability Theory

Generalizability Theory uses the concept of generalizability instead of reliability, considering observed scores to be a sample of possible scores (Streiner and Norman, 1989; Cronbach *et al*, 1972). GT establishes how accurately observed scores can be generalized to a defined universe of scores. Different sources of error - facets - define the universe of scores, such as individuals, time of measurement, and health state. Each facet consists of different conditions, for example 'respondent 1' and 'respondent 5' for the facet 'individuals', 'time TEST' and 'time RETEST' for the facet 'time of measurement', health state '11211' and '33333' for the facet 'health state'.

An application of GT is a Generalizability Study (G-study). A G-study estimates empirically the variance of facets (variance components) of a given universe of scores. It is carried out by means of an analysis of variance, in which an estimation of variance for each facet is obtained from the expected mean squares. For our G-study we used the BMDP computer programme (subroutine 8V), in which the estimation of the variance components are derived from the Cornfield and Tukey formulae (1956). The resulting estimated variance components are used to calculate the contribution of each source of variability relative to total variance.

In our study variances for three main sources of variances were estimated, namely PERSON (P), TIME (T), HEALTH STATE (H), to which 4 interactions were added: PT, PH, TH and PTH, which includes also (by definition) all other unknown error variance. A G-study was applied to all 4 versions of the questionnaire.

9.4 RESULTS

Response

The response characteristics per version of the questionnaire are given in Table 9.2. The general response rate for the study on test-retest reliability amounted to 302 of the total of 398 (75%). Qf these, 208 were usable for analysis (defined as less than 2 valuations missing, plus consistency).

Table 9.2 Response per version of the questionnaire

	Version of the questionnaire				
	AB	CB	AD	CD	Total
Total addressed	86	110	97	105	398
Total response	69	61	84	88	302
Usable*	56	47	61	67	231
Usable and consistent **	52	40	56	60	208

* <= 2 valuations missing
** health state 11111 > health state 33333

Background characteristics

Differences in background characteristics between the usable and consistent respondents of both the Rotterdam Survey and the test-retest sample, some of which are shown in Table 9.3, were not statistically significant according to the two-sided t-test. We concluded the second sample to be representative of the first.

Table 9.3 Relevant background characteristics of respondents: total sample (only first survey) and test-retest sample (first and second survey)

	Usable and consistent response 1st survey N = 596	Usable and consistent response 1st and 2nd survey N = 208	p
Sex (% women)	43.3	43.3	
Age (Years)	X = 47.7 SD = 18.3 Md = 44.0	X = 49.3 SD = 18.1 Md = 46.5	.284
Valuation of own health (0 = 'worst imaginable health state'; 100 = best imaginable health state)	X = 81.4 SD = 14.6 Md = 85.0	X = 82.6 SD = 13.8 Md = 85.0	.322

Valuations

The mean and median valuations in test and retest are shown in Table 9.4. Apparently the mean valuations of test and retest are in the same range. In addition the tendency of smaller standard deviations for the descriptions of 'extreme' health states ('11111' and '33333'), as a result of the end-point position of these health states on the health status scale, is apparent on both occasions.

Table 9.4 Valuations in test and retest (n = 208)

	TEST			RETEST		
State	X	SD	Md	X	SD	Md
11111a	94.1	11.3	98	95.0	7.2	98
11111b	94.6	8.7	98	94.4	8.7	98
11211	80.5	11.8	80	82.0	11.2	85
11121	74.5	15.7	75	74.6	14.9	79
11112	73.2	15.3	75	72.9	15.3	74.5
12111	70.2	19.7	75	72.3	15.8	75
21111	66.0	17.6	70	64.4	18.0	65
11221	66.1	15.5	70	65.0	15.6	65
11122	59.4	16.8	60	62.0	15.4	60
21211	53.9	20.8	60	51.2	20.6	50
12212	52.8	17.3	52	55.0	18.4	55
21212	47.3	17.1	50	44.1	16.6	45
32211	44.0	17.9	45	42.3	17.2	42
21232	31.6	17.7	30	35.1	17.0	35
2322.3	25.4	16.9	25	25.7	16.9	25
22233	23.4	15.3	20	25.5	14.3	22
33321	23.8	16.0	20	22.6	12.6	21
22323	22.5	16.1	20	22.5	14.5	20
22333	21.0	18.6	15	20.6	16.0	15
32233	20.6	18.2	19	20.1	16.3	17.5
23332	18.2	16.0	15	17.0	14.8	15
32333	16.0	16.5	10	15.6	13.2	10
33233	15.7	15.1	10	15.5	11.3	14
33332	16.1	14.0	15	17.0	14.6	15
23333	11.7	13.1	9.5	10.9	10.3	10
uncons*	10.1	17.3	3	12.1	18.2	5
33333a	8.1	12.7	5	8.8	10.4	5
33333b	8.5	11.6	5	8.4	10.0	5

* unconscious

The two MDU approaches, assuming respectively ordinal and interval character of the valuation data, showed almost the same results, as indicated by equal values of the measure of badness-of-fit, the stress - approximately 0,2 (according to Young's S-stress formula 2 [Torgerson, 1958]) - and the resulting coordinates of the health states onto the underlying continuum, which are graphically displayed in Figure 9.2. These results imply that the scale, taking into account the information from all individual valuations, has the characteristics of an interval scale, such as equi-distancy. Hence the assumption of interval scaled valuations is justified if the respondents are considered as a group as we accomplished in subsequent analyses.

Figure 9.2 shows that the slopes of both curves of the two sets of MDU scale values follow the slope of the curve of the mean valuations quite closely, apart from a deviation at health state 'unconscious'. Hence the underlying scale is appropriately represented by the observed mean valuations.

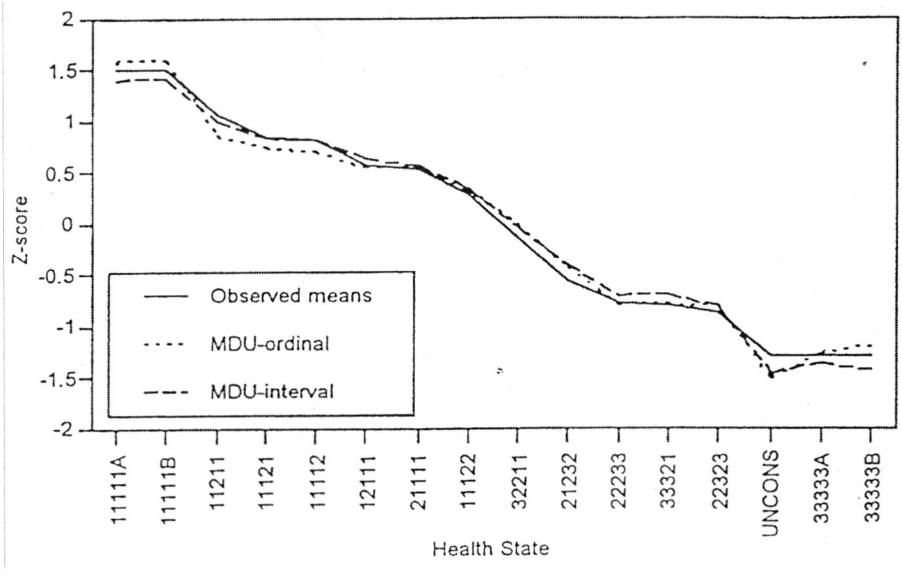

Figure 9.2 Values (z-scores) of health state valuations
(first moment of measurement of version AB: n=52):
Observed mean valuations and MDU scaled valuations, assuming respectively ordinal (MDU-ordinal) and interval data (MDU-interval)

Further investigations revealed that this deviation was caused by 4 'outlier' respondents who ranked/valued the health state 'unconscious' among the best states of the set. (These outliers were not omitted from further analysis).

Test-retest reliability

Generalizability Study: the results of the G-study are shown in Table 9.5, which presents estimated variance components and percentages of variance to total variance for each version of the questionnaire. The results per version appear to be very similar. Almost all variance is attributed to the variability of HEALTH STATE scores (77% to 84%). Eight to twelve percent of total variance comes from the three-way interaction PTH, which also includes all unexplained error. The interpretation of this interaction term is: there may be some respondents who value some health states very differently the first or the second time. The component TIME and interaction component TH have zero or negligible variances; in addition the interaction PT is relatively small (1% - 4%). The relative contribution to total variability of PERSON (ranging from 1% to 3%) indicates that, averaged over time of measurement and over all health states, respondents value health states slightly differently. This also holds for PH (4% - 5%), i.e. averaged over time of measurement minor differences exist between valuations of some respondents for particular health states.

Table 9.5 Results of the Generalizability Study per version of the questionnaire

Source of variation	Estimated variance component			
	Version AB	Version CB	Version AD	Version CD
Person	33.9	23.4	15.7	28.3
Time	0.6	0.0	0.0	0.0
Health state	966.5	795.6	974.4	924.5
PT	15.4	43.5	25.7	37.5
PH	51.3	44.1	54.6	64.1
Th	1.4	0.0	0.4	0.0
Pm	110.0	126.0	89.8	122.1
Total	1179.2	1032.6	1160.6	1176.5

Source of variation	Percentage to total variance			
	Version AB	Version CB	Version AD	Version CD
Person	2.87%	2.27%	1.35%	2.41%
Time	0.05%	0%	0%	0%
Health state	81.96%	77.05%	83.96%	78.58%
PT	1.31%	4.21%	2.21%	3.19%
PH	4.35%	4.27%	4.70%	5.45%
Th	0.12%	0%	0.03%	0%
Pm	9.33%	12.20%	7.74%	10.38%
Total	100%	100%	100%	100%

9.5 CONCLUSION AND DISCUSSION

This study aimed at establishing reliability of the valuation of health states, using the EuroQol measurement procedure. As three sources of variances had to be analyzed simultaneously (test-retest variability, variability due to individual responses, and variability due to the different health states to be valued), a statistical approach was chosen which goes beyond classical test theory and conventional ANOVA. The suitable approach following Cronbach (1972), and Streiner and Norman (1989) appears to be G-theory, an ANOVA-based technique. However, this technique required us to investigate the nature (measurement level) of the data. Before we discuss the results on reliability, some remarks will be presented on the preceding methodological steps. Comparison of the aspirations and requirements of existing techniques, and of the available standard computer packages, showed that an ordinal measurement level gives rise to important analytical restrictions, whereas in the case of interval data the application of more sophisticated ANOVA-models requires manual computations based on ANOVA-output.

The results of ALSCAL for determination of the measurement level of the valuation data were surprising: the EuroQol valuations could be validly regarded as interval scores. In the context of the application of these values in economic evaluation, this accidental finding is very important. Many aggregation procedures, *inter alia* the calculation of Quality Adjusted Life Years (QALYs), depend on the measurement level of the valuation data. This is the first evidence on this issue which favours the assumption of interval properties for these valuations. Of course this result should be confirmed, preferably using another classification such as the Quality of Well-Being scale (Kaplan et al, 1976), to allow for valid generalizations on this topic.

As a final methodological result we conclude that G-theory offers a feasible method to summarize test-retest data if multiple independent variables and multiple sources of variance exist. In this G-study, the valuations of the 16 health states of each version of the questionnaire were analysed coherently, while several sources of variance (health states, respondents, and moment of measurement) could be accounted for in one analysis.

The preceding steps all contributed to the firm conclusion that valuations are stable over time. Only .05% of variance for valuations in version AB (standard EuroQol) of the questionnaire is explained by the systematic effect of the facet TIME. This percentage should be related to the other sources of variance, the most important in this case being 82% for HEALTH STATE, and 10% for the interaction term PTH. Probably the largest contribution of the facet TIME exists in this interaction component. This cannot be proved however, because the highest order interaction component cannot make a distinction between real PTH interaction and all other unexplained error. So theoretically the maximal contribution of TIME is TIME + PT + TH + PTH, which amounted to at most eleven percent. This percentage of variance explained by the total variance of TIME is low compared to the 82% explained by HEALTH STATE. Hence, we concluded that test-retest reliability for version AB is good. The fact that this finding was confirmed for the other versions of the questionnaire, which for this purpose may be regarded as independent replicating samples, reinforces this conclusion.

It can be argued that the results are flattered because by far the largest percentage of variance is caused by the facet HEALTH STATE. This source of variation is imposed by the questionnaire. If HEALTH STATE is neglected as a source of variance, approximately 50% of the remaining variance is caused by PTH and 25% by PH. The contribution of TIME again remains very small and is only detectable in PTH (which includes, by definition, all other error).

We found only one study in the medical literature dealing with test-retest reliability of a rating scale for valuations of health states with a long interval. Torrance reported a one-year test-retest reliability with a rating scale of .49 (correlation coefficient) (Torrance, 1976). His article, however, does not clarify whether this is a coefficient at the group-level calculated for each health state and averaged over health states, or a coefficient derived from individual correlations considering all health states simultaneously. For our study, the comparable figure is .36 for the former, and .90 for the latter. It should be noted that Torrance excluded health states from the calculations when respondents stated afterwards that they had altered their attitude towards these states. It is very likely that this selection influenced the test-retest reliability coefficient favourably.

The time interval chosen in the present study was 10 months. Generally, the time interval for test-retest studies should be both long enough to exclude recollection effects, and short enough to exclude changes in the characteristics under study. Recollection effects for the EuroQol valuation questionnaire can safely be considered to be non-existent after 10 months. The only characteristic known from the literature to influence valuations of health states to any relevant extent is a person's own health state. In the second survey respondents were asked if their health state had changed since the first survey. Their responses reveal that the health state of 80% of all respondents had not experienced a change during the last ten months. Exclusion of the respondents who indicated that their health state had changed, did not alter the results significantly.

To conclude: the establishment of the test-retest reliability of the EuroQol valuations demonstrates the EuroQol's success in carefully developing a two-stage measuring instrument for describing and valuing health status. It contributes also to the completion of the uniquely defined aim of the EuroQol to establish all psychometric properties of its instrument.

9.6 ACKNOWLEDGEMENTS

The authors wish to thank Marlies E.A. Stouthard MSc PhD and Maurice Palmen BSc for their assistance with this study.

Presented at the EuroQol Plenary Meeting: Helsinki, Finland, 1992

9.7 REFERENCES

Bergner M, Bobitt R A, et al. The Sickness Impact Profile: Conceptual formulation and methodology for the development of a health status measure. Int. J. of Health Services 1976;6:393-415.

Brooks R G, Jendteg S, Lindgren B, Persson U, Björk S. EuroQol: health-related quality of life measurement. results of the Swedish questionnaire exercise. Health Policy 1991;18:37-48.

Cornfield J, Tukey J W. Average values of mean squares in factorials. Ann. Math. Statist. 1956;27:907-949.

Cronbach L J, Gleser G C, Nanda H, Rajaratnam N. The dependability of behavioral measurements: Theory of generalizability of scores and profiles. Wiley, New York, 1972.

Essink-Bot M L, Bonsel G J, Maas P J van der. Valuation of health states by the general public: feasibility of a standardized measurement procedure. Soc. Sci. Med. 1990;31:1201-1206.

Essink-Bot M L, Stouthard M E A, Bonsel G J. Generalizability of valuations on health states collected with the EuroQol-questionnaire. Health Economics 1993;2:237-247.

EuroQol Group. EuroQol - a new facility for the measurement of health-related quality of life. Health Policy 1990;16:199-208.

EuroQol Group. EuroQol - A reply and reminder. Health Policy 1992a;20:329-332.

EuroQol Group. EuroQol Conference Proceedings 1991. Björk S, editor. IHE Working Paper 1992:2. Lund: Institute for Health Economics, 1992b.

EuroQol Group. EuroQol Conference Proceedings 1992. Sintonen H, editor. Discussion Paper No 2. Kuopio: Department of Social Sciences, 1993.

Goombs G H. Psychological scaling without a unit of measurement. Psychol. Rev. 1950;57:145-158.

Hunt S M, McEwen J, Mckenna S P. Measuring Health Status, London: Croom Helm, 1986.

Kaplan R M, Bush J W, Berry C C. Health status: Types of validity for an index of well-being. Health Serv. Res. 1976;11;478-507.

Nord E. EuroQol: health-related quality of life measurement. valuations of health states by the general public in Norway. Health Policy 1991;18:25-36.

Rosser R, Sintonen H. The EuroQol quality of life project. In: Walker S R, Rosser R M, editors. Quality of Life: Key issues in 1990s. Kluwer Academic Publishers, 1993:197-198.

Streiner D, Norman G R. Health measurement scales: a practical guide to their development and use. Oxford University Press, 1989.

Siegel S, Castellan J N. Nonparametric statistics for the behavioral sciences. 2nd Edition. McGraw-Hill Book Company, 1988.

Takane Y, Young F, Leeuw J de. Nonmetric individual differences multidimensional scaling: an alternating least square method with optimal scaling features. Psychometrika 1977;42:7-67.

Torgerson W S. Theory and methods of scaling. John Wiley and Sons, Inc., 1958.

Torrance G W. Social preferences for health states: an empirical evaluation of three measurement techniques. Soclo-Econ. Plan. Sci. 1976;10:129-136.

10
Hypothetical valuations of health states versus patients' self-ratings

Erik Nord, Xavier Badia, Montserrat Rue and Harri Sintonen

10.1 INTRODUCTION

Health status indices are tools for informing clinical decisions and resource allocation. Most of today's indices, including the EuroQol, are based on valuations of health states by samples of the general population. The subjects are asked to imagine themselves in different states of illness and to indicate the degree of disutility they think they would experience in each of these states. A serious concern that arises from this research is whether people can be expected to know what it is like to be in health states that they have never experienced (Selai and Rosser, 1995).

Defenders of hypothetical valuations may argue that the descriptive systems of health status index instruments are not in terms of diagnoses, but rather in terms of concrete symptoms and functional impairments. The subjects need therefore not be familiar with specific illnesses. They only need to know the disutility of such health problems as not being able to walk, work or dress etc or of having pain, nausea, sleeplessness etc. Arguably, these are dysfunctions which most people are able to judge on the basis of personal experience some time in their life.

The problem, however, is the time factor. Clinical decision-making and resource allocation decisions are largely about helping patients with chronic or potentially chronic conditions. The impact on quality of life of long-lasting but stable dysfunctions may be quite different from the effects of temporary disruptive illness episodes experienced by otherwise healthy people. The difference may go both ways. On the one hand, patients may become mentally worn out and increasingly frustrated by long-lasting illness (Sutherland *et al*, 1982). On the other hand, chronically ill people may learn over time to adjust their expectations and to cope with situations that at first seem difficult or hopeless (Calman, 1984).

This does not mean that hypothetical valuations are useless. Policy-makers will to some extent have to accommodate the beliefs of the general population - be they right or wrong - when making decisions about resource allocation. Hypothetical valuations are also easy to elicit in large numbers and therefore constitute a relatively quick way to gain some commonsense based insight into the disutility of different kinds of illness. However, hypothetical valuations cannot be the whole story. In monitoring health, and in clinical decision-making, patients' actual perceptions of the disutility of illness must clearly be more relevant than the general population's beliefs about

P. Kind et al. (eds.), EQ-5D concepts and methods, 125–138.

illness. And in resource allocation decisions, it would be irrational for decision-makers to place great emphasis on the general populations' beliefs if they had reason to think that the beliefs deviated significantly from reality, but also we must assume that the general population's beliefs would change if it turned out that the patients themselves felt differently and this was communicated to people in general.

In the appendix to this paper (10.1) we review some previously published studies on quality of life in people with illness. In the main text we present data from the Finnish and the Catalan EuroQol surveys that show how people in different EuroQol states rate their own quality of life. We compare these self-ratings with the scores obtained for the same states when valued hypothetically by all the subjects in the surveys. Unfortunately the comparison is justified only at an ordinal level of measurement, and there are only a few states that are covered both by hypothetical valuations and self-ratings. This part of the paper must therefore be seen as strictly exploratory. In a final section we shed some light on the York TTO tariff by comparing it very briefly with TTO results from non-EuroQol patient studies.

10.2 SUMMARY OF PREVIOUS LITERATURE

While the studies reviewed in the appendix provide neither an accurate nor an exhaustive picture of quality of life in patients, some tentative conclusions may be drawn. First, the quality of life associated with a given condition varies widely. Second, chronically ill people seem to differ less from healthy people in terms of subjectively perceived well-being than one might expect by simply judging health differences. Third, the expressed disutility and the willingness to sacrifice (longevity) to be relieved of illness seem somewhat less when patients are asked to evaluate their own current health state than when healthy people are asked to evaluate different hypothetical conditions. The ability to cope and to adapt to illness over time presents itself as a likely explanation for all these observations.

10.3 EUROQOL DATA

Hypothetical valuations in the EuroQol are mainly scores on a visual analogue scale. These valuations may be compared with self-ratings that people in different states have given on the same scale. The York Group has also elicited hypothetical valuations by means of the time trade-off technique. There are no TTO-based self-ratings of EuroQol states with which these hypothetical valuations can be compared. There are at least three problems with comparisons of hypothetical visual analogue scale scores with self-ratings.

First, there is a contextual difference between the two valuation tasks. In the hypothetical part, eight states are valued at a time on the same scale. To allow sufficient separation between all these states, responders may need to utilize the full range of the scale, in other words to locate 11111 close to the upper end and the worst states close to the lower end. In the self-rating exercise, on the other hand, "best imaginable" and "worst imaginable" are the only reference points. Respondents presumably feel that their own state, however good or bad it is, should be located at some distance from these extremes. We would therefore expect greater compression towards the middle in the self-rating responses than in the hypothetical ones.

In theory, this difference in the use of the scale could be accounted for by transform ing the values in both the hypothetical and the self-rating sets to a scale where state 11111 was assigned 100 and the state "dead" was assigned 0. In practice this is not possible, since the state "dead", for understandable reasons, was not covered by responses to the self-rating scale on page 3. Possibly some severe state could be chosen in stead of "dead" as a bottom anchoring point. This possibility is being explored by the Spanish Group.

Second, there is a potential heterogeneity bias. When subjects describe themselves on page 2, people with quite different symptom levels may be forced into the same crude categories. For instance, among those who describe themselves as being in state 21111, some probably have only slight problems with walking, while others may be wheelchair users. On page 3, we must assume that they consider the actual intensity of their problems rather than the levels they were forced to choose in the crude "menu" on page 2. The mean of the VAS-ratings in those classified as 21111 is therefore really the mean in a group with a distribution around 21111. If the distribution is symmetrical, there is no difference between this group mean and the mean one would find in a group of people for whom the description "some problems" was really adequate. However, there are two factors which could lead to the distribution being asymmetrical. The two factors work in opposite ways. On the one hand, slight problems (less than "some problems") are more common in the survey sample than considerable problems (more than "some problems"). This implies that the group of subjects forced into category 21111 could on average have less than "some problems". On the other hand, in field studies with the EuroQol Instrument the lack of a level between present levels 2 and 3 has much more often been reported as a problem than the lack of a level between present levels 1 and 2. This is true of all dimensions, but particularly of mobility, where there is a leap from "some problems" to "bedridden". This means that the size of the error associated with those who are forced to choose level 2 from "below" (from a real level between 2 and 3) is likely to be greater than the error associated with those who are forced from "above" (from between level 1 and 2). This again implies that the real level of problems with walking in the 21111-group could be greater than that indicated by the label "some problems".

The net effect of the two factors mentioned here is difficult to assess. It does however leave us with the following problem: Assume that subjects evaluate, say, state 21111 hypothetically. When doing so, they take into consideration the phrase "some problems with walking". We then compare their evaluations with the self-ratings of people who are registered as having "some problems with walking", but who on average may actually have problems that should be described in either weaker or stronger terms. The hypothetical valuation and the self-rating would then not be comparable.

Third, there is a potential comprehensiveness bias. When subjects rate themselves on page 3, we must assume that they also take into account symptoms and dysfunctions that are not covered by the EuroQol descriptive system (for instance nausea or allergic reaction). Such other problems are implicitly presented as non-existent in the hypothetical valuation exercise. This means that self-ratings on page 3 tend to refer to more severe states than corresponding hypothetical valuations, even if the 5-digit codes are the same in both cases.

Given these biases, we find it difficult at present to compare self-ratings and hypothetical valuations on the EuroQol visual analogue scale at a cardinal level of measurement. That is, we are not sure that the visual analogue scale data allow us to judge whether quality of life in patients is higher (or lower) than indicated by hypothetical valuations. However, it is possible to ascertain the weights that are implicitly assigned to the five different dimensions of health in the hypothetical valuations and to see whether these are supported by the weights that emerge from the self-ratings. This is our aim in the following sections, where we draw on data from the Finnish and the Catalan EuroQol studies.

Contextual bias is less of a problem in time trade-off exercises, where states are valued separately one by one. A comparison of the hypothetical TTO-valuations elicited by the York Group with TTO-based self-ratings of the same states might therefore be justified in cardinal terms. However, as noted above, such self-ratings do not exist at the moment. In a final section we confine ourselves to shedding some light on the York TTO tariff by comparing it very briefly with the previously mentioned TTO results from non-EuroQol patient studies.

10.4 THE FINNISH EUROQOL STUDY

In the main Finnish EuroQol study, conducted in 1993, eleven different versions were made of the EuroQol questionnaire. Each version used the same standard wording, but the set of hypothetical states to be valued varied. Each version was mailed to a random population sample of 230 people. Altogether 2530 questionnaires were distributed. 1650 were returned. Of these, 1003 were usable, yielding a net response rate of 40%.

586 respondents were in state 11111. There were twelve other states in which there were at least five repondents. Table 10.1 shows the mean self-rating of these respon-

dents on the visual analogue scale. Eight of these states were valued hypothetically by all responders in the second part of the questionnaire. Table 10.1 also shows the means of these valuations.

Table 10.1 Self-ratings and hypothetical valuations in the Finnish EuroQol study

	Self-rating			Hypothetical valuation		
State	Mean	SE	N	Mean	SE	N
11111	89	0.4	586	96	0.2	999
21111	82	1.5	11	78	0.6	577
11112	80	1.6	40	62	0.9	578
11121	80	1.1	136	75	0.7	531
11122	76	2.7	33	47	0.8	529
11211	75	3.0	7	79	0.6	528
21121	73	2.6	33			
21122	68	4.6	8			
11221	68	3.6	11			
11222	65	6.7	8			
21221	62	2.1	38			
21222	57	4.0	14	36	1.2	188
22221	55	4.3	14	44	1.3	166

As can be seen, there are particularly large differences for states including a negative score on the mood dimension (11112, 11122, 21222). A possible explanation may be that people do not regard mood as an equally obvious dimension of health as the other four dimensions of the EuroQol (A similar point has previously been made regarding the Rosser/Kind index, see Nord, 1992). On page 3 of the questionnaire, where there is reference to "health" only, respondents may therefore tend to give little weight to mood (anxiety/depression). In the hypothetical valuation task, on the other hand, subjects are encouraged to include mood in the concept of health as it is explicitly included as a dimension in each box.

If this is correct, then self-ratings and hypothetical valuations in the EuroQol exercise refer to different concepts. The scores are then compatible only with states where mood is at level one.

In Table 10.1 there are only five states that satisfy this condition, for which there are both self-ratings and hypothetical valuations. One may note that according to self-ratings, a drop to level 2 on the usual activity dimension (11211) means more than a corresponding drop on the pain dimension (11121), while subjects thought the opposite in the hypothetical context.

Table 10.2 shows the results of regressing mean hypothetical valuations and mean VAS self-ratings, respectively, on the five health dimensions. While mood is the dimension with the strongest partial effect in hypothetical valuations, it is one of the two with the smallest effect in self-ratings. As noted above, this could be due to differences in framing rather than an expression of real differences between hypothetical valuations and self-ratings. On the other hand, usual activity has the strongest partial effect in self-ratings, while it has the smallest effect in hypothetical valuations. This corresponds to the observation of the values of states 11211 and 11121 in the previous paragraph and might be an example of hypothetical valuations not capturing the real experience of patients.

Table 10.2 Regression of hypothetical valuations and self-ratings on health dimensions

	Hypothetical valuations		Self-ratings	
Variable	B	SE	B	SE
Mobility	-9.2	1.5	-7.2	1.3
Self-care	-6.2	1.7	-9.4	1.8
Usual activity	-5.4	1.6	-11.2	1.3
Pain	-7.7	1.5	-8.3	0.9
Mood	-9.3	1.5	-7.4	1.1
Constant	114.2	4.4	131.8	1.8
	$R^2 = 0.88$		$R^2 = 0.52$	

10.5 THE CATALAN EUROQOL STUDY

In Catalonia, the standard EuroQol Instrument was used to collect valuations of 15 health states from 600 individuals attending a primary care center, 120 chronic patients, and 103 critically ill patients (Badia *et al*, 1995).

In the 1994 Catalan health survey the EuroQol was included as one of the survey questionnaires. 15000 subjects were interviewed. For people under 15 years of age and people unable to answer, responses were obtained from proxies. These individuals are excluded in the present analysis. Self-ratings by means of the EuroQol Instrument were obtained for 12055 individuals. To obtain a wider range of health states, data on the 120 chronic patients and 103 critically ill patients mentioned above are included in the present study, resulting in a sample of 12278 subjects for which we have self-ratings. 8147 subjects were in state 11111. There were 37 other states in which there were at least 10 respondents. Table 10.3 shows the mean self-rating of these respondents on the visual analogue scale.

Table 10.3 Self-ratings in the Catalan EuroQol study

	Self-rating				Self-rating		
State	Mean	SD	N	State	Mean	SD	N
11111	77	14	8147	21122	51	13	102
12111	69	19	10	21131	50	17	58
11211	67	17	41	21212	50	11	11
11112	66	16	403	22221	50	17	39
11121	66	16	1351	21231	49	15	41
21111	62	17	171	11231	48	27	13
11113	59	18	54	21132	47	21	41
21211	59	19	33	11222	46	17	43
11122	58	15	372	22232	46	18	18
21121	56	16	348	21222	45	16	75
21112	56	16	26	22222	44	17	27
11221	56	20	70	21123	44	12	17
12221	56	12	11	11133	43	21	25
11123	55	16	40	21232	41	16	56
11132	55	16	60	11232	39	13	14
11131	54	18	104	33322	39	15	12
21221	54	17	113	21233	33	15	24
22211	52	15	13	11233	31	16	10
11212	51	18	11	22233	23	11	11

Eleven of the 15 states that were valued hypothetically in the first study occurred at least 5 times in the ensuing health survey. Table 10.4 shows self-ratings and hypothetical valuations for these states. We may note that according to the hypothetical valuations, having some problems with self-care (12111) is distinctly worse than having some problems along any of the other four dimensions. This finding does not stand up in the self-ratings. The hypothetical valuations of the three poorest states are also very different from the corresponding self-ratings both in terms of rank ordering and absolute scores. Subjects seem to have attached more importance to the first three dimensions than to the last two in the hypothetical valuations (see state 33321, which scores 12, versus 21232 and 22233, which score 37 and 25). In the self-ratings, by contrast, state 33321 for example scores twice as high as 22233.

Table 10.4 Self-ratings and hypothetical valuations in the Catalan EuroQol study

State	Self-ratings Mean	SE	N	Hypothetical valuations Mean (N=823, se=0.3-0.7)
11111	77	0.2	8147	98
12111	69	6.0	10	57
11211	67	2.7	41	72
11112	66	0.8	403	76
11121	66	0.4	1351	76
21111	62	1.3	171	73
11122	58	0.8	372	55
22322	53	7.9	6	32
33321	46	6.7	9	12
21232	41	2.0	56	37
22233	23	3.3	11	25

10.6 THE YORK TIME TRADE-OFF TARIFF

The York time trade-off tariff (Williams, 1995) is based on interviews with a representative sample of 3000 non-institutionalized adults in England, Scotland and Wales. Each subject valued 15 different states. Altogether 45 states were valued, most by approximately 800 subjects. Values for those states that were not included in the study were later estimated by regressing the observed scores on the five EuroQol dimensions of health. The value structure of the tariff may be indicated as follows:

(i)	Some problems on only one of the five EuroQol dimensions (mobility, self-care, usual activity, pain, anxiety/depression):	0.80-0.88
(ii)	Some problems on two dimensions:	0.70-0.80
(iii)	Some problems on three dimensions:	0.60-0.70
(iv)	Very severe problems on only one dimension:	0.25-0.55

By comparison, Churchill *et al* (1984) found a TTO score of 0.54 in hamodialysis patients. Tsevat found a mean score of 0.73 in very seriously ill patients confronted with a one year life perspective. Fryback *et al* (1993) suggest scores between 0.75 and 0.85 for patients with insulin dependent diabetes, depression, asthma and chronic bronchitis and scores between 0.90 and 0.95 in people with arthritis, severe back pain, migraine, angina, cataract, ulcer, colitis, and sleep disorder.

These results leave us with the impression that patients are in reality less willing to sacrifice longevity to become well than is suggested by the hypothetical valuations obtained by the York Group.

10.7 CONCLUSION

The literature on quality of life in people with illness suggests that the chronically ill differ less from healthy people in terms of subjectively perceived well-being than one might expect by simply judging health differences. In particular, the expressed disutility and the willingness to sacrifice (longevity) to be relieved of illness seem somewhat less when patients are asked to evaluate their own current health state than when healthy people are asked to evaluate different hypothetical conditions. The present study suggests that this bias in hypothetical valuations may also be a problem in the EuroQol enterprise. To determine the magnitude of the problem, time trade-off based self-ratings of EuroQol states would be particularly valuable. Such data could serve to develop a full tariff of patients' valuations of EuroQol states.

Presented at the EuroQol Plenary Meeting: Barcelona, Spain, 1995

10.8 REFERENCES

Aaronson N K. Methodologic issues in assessing the quality of life of cancer patients. Cancer 1991;67:844-850.

Badia X, et al. Influence of socio-demographic and health status variables on evaluation of health states in a Spanish population. European Journal of Public Health 1995;5:87-93.

Bombardier C, et al. Comparison of three preference measurement methodologies in the evaluation of a functional status index. In: Deber R B, Thompson G G, editors. Choice in Health Care. University of Toronto: Dept of Health Admin, 1982.

Buxton M, Ashby J, O'Hanlon M. Alternative methods of valuing health states. Mimeo. Brunel University: HERG, 1987.

Calman K C. Quality of life in cancer patients - an hypothesis. Journal of Medical Ethics 1984;10:124-127.

Cassileth B R, et al. Psychosocial status in chronic illness. A comparative analysis of six diagnostic groups. New England Journal of Medicine 1984;311:506-511.

Churchill D N, Morgan J, Torrance G W. Quality of life in end stage renal disease. Peritoneal Dialysis Bulletin 1984;Jan-March:20- 23.

Clipp E C, Elder G H. Elderly confidants in geriatric assessment. Compr Gerontol B 1987;1:35-40.

Derogatis L R, Abeloff M D, McBeth C D. Cancer patients and their physicians in the perception of psychological symptoms. Psychosomatics 1976;17:197-201.

Epstein A M, et al. Using proxies to evaluate quality of life. Medical Care 1989;27:S91-S98.

Fryback D G, Dasbach E J, Klein R, et al. The beaver dam health outcomes study. Medical Decision Making 1993;13:89-102.

Knussen C, Cunningham C C. Stress, disability and handicap. In: Fisher S, Reason J, editors. Handbook of life stress. Wiley and Sons Ltd, 1988.

Llewellyn-Thomas H A, Sutherland H J, Thiel E. Do patients' evaluations of a future health state change when they actually enter that stage? Med Care 1993;31:1002-1012.

Magaziner J, Simonsick E M, Kashner T M, Hebel J R. Patient-proxy response comparability on measures of patient health and functional status. Journal of Clinical Epidemiology 1988;41:1065-1074.

McCusker J, Stoddard A M. Use of a surrogate for the sickness impact profile. Medical Care 1984;22:789-795.

Nord E. Bedømming av pasienters livskvalitet. (Assessing patients' quality of life. A literature review.) Forskningsrapport nr. Fl-1992. Oslo: Statens institutt for folkehelse, seksjon for helsetjenesteforskning, 1992.

O'Brien J, Francis A. The use of next-of-kin to estimate pain in cancer patients. Pain 1988;35:171-178.

Pearlman R A, Uhlmann R F. Quality of life in chronic diseases: Perceptions of elderly patients. Journal of Gerontology 1988;43(M2):5-30.

Read J L, et al. Prefererences for health outcomes. Comparison of assessment methods. Med Decis Making 1984;4:315-329.

Richardson J, Hall J, Salkeld G. Cost utility analysis: The compatibility of measurement techniques and the measurement of utility through time. In: Smith C S, editor. Economics and health. Proceedings of the Eleventh Australian Conference of Health Economists, 1989.

Rothman M L et al. The validity of proxy-generated scores as measures of patient health status. Medical Care 1991;29:115-124.

Rubinstein L Z, Schairer C, Wieland G D, Kane R. Systematic biases in functional status assessment of elderly adults: Effects of different data sources. J of Gerontology, 1984;39:686-691.

Selai C, Rosser R. Eliciting EuroQol descriptive data and utility scale values from inpatients. Pharmacoeconomics 1995;8:147-158.

Slevin M L, et al. Who should measure quality of life, the doctor or the patient? British Journal of Cancer 1988;57:109-112.

Spitzer W O, et al. Measuring the quality of life in cancer patients. Journal of Chronical Disease 1981;34:585-597.

Stewart A, et al. Functional status and well-being of patients with chronic conditions. JAMA, 1989, 262, 907-913.

Sutherland H J, Llewellyn-Thomas H, Boyd N F, Till J E. Attitudes toward quality of survival. The concept of "maximum endurable time". Medical Decision Making 1982;2:299-309.

Tsevat J, et al. Health values of the seriously ill. Annals of Internal Medicine 1994;122:514-520.

Williams A. The measurement and valuation of health: A chronicle. Discussion paper 136. York: Centre for Health Economics, 1995.

Yager J, Linn L S. Physician-patient agreement about depression: Notation in medical records. General Hospital Psychiatry 1981;3:271-276.

APPENDIX 10.1

STUDIES OF QUALITY OF LIFE IN PATIENTS

The variability in the way in which illness affects quality of life is indicated in a study by Spitzer *et al* (1981). These authors used the Quality of Life Index to score (a) a group of mainly healthy people who consulted general practitioners for trivial or temporary conditions, (b) patients with severe chronic diseases such as rheumatoid arthritis, advanced diabetes, spinal injury or chronic obstructive lung disease, (c) patients with the most common kinds of cancer, and (d) critically- or terminally-ill patients.

The instrument includes the following dimensions: activity (employment, studying, housework), everyday life (moving about and self-care), health (self-assessed feeling of being healthy), support (support from and contact with family and friends), and outlook (anxiety/depression). Each dimension has three steps (0/1/2), so that the maximum total score is 10. The healthy had a mean score of 9.0, versus 7.3 in the chronically ill, 7.1 in the cancer patients, and 3.3 in the critically ill. Interestingly, however, 18% of the chronically ill obtained the maximum score (10) in spite of the severity of their condition. More than half scored 8 or higher, while 25% scored 5 or lower. Similar figures were found for the cancer patients. By contrast, in the critically- or terminally-ill, 80% of the patients scored 4 or less.

Cassileth *et al* (1984) examined 758 patients with arthritis, depression, diabetes, cancer, terminal renal failure and skin disease by means of the Mental Health Index. The Index has 43 items, and the patients are scored on a scale from zero to one hundred with respect to anxiety, depression, positive affect, emotional ties, loss of control and global mental health. On all these dimensions, mental health was found to be 10-15 percentage points higher in 60-years olds than in 40-year olds in the six patient groups in question. The authors suggest that "chronic illness, ironically, offers social advantages that are less available to the healthy elderly, such as increases in activity, involvement with others, and the amount of attention and concern received. On the basis of years and experience, older people may develop more effective skills with which to manage stressful life events. Their perspective and expectations may be more commensurate with adaptation to illness than is the case for younger patients. There may be a biological, evolutionary advantage for older patients, enabling them to adapt to illnesses that are epidemiologically associated with advancing years" (p.509).

Pearlman and Uhlmann (1988) studied 126 patients over 64 years old with at least one of the following chronic diseases: arthritis, ischaemic heart disease, chronic lung disease, diabetes mellitus, and cancer. Patients described their global quality of life on a 6-step scale ranging from "about as good as possible" to "terrible, quality of life is very poor". Differences between mean scores in the different patient groups were very small (means ranged from 2.1 to 2.4) and were statistically non-significant, in spite of the large differences in the illnesses themselves. On average, the patients described their own health as somewhere between "good" and "fair", judged their health to be a little better than "average for most people of the same sex and age", and felt that their health problems affected their quality of life only a little more than "slightly".

Stewart *et al* (1989) examined (a) 5068 patients spread over 9 chronic diseases (hypertension, diabetes, heart failure, myocardiac infarction, arthritis, chronic lung disease, gastrointestinal disease, back pain and angina), (b) 2595 non-chronically ill patients, and (c) 2002 people from the general population, using the Medical Outcomes Study Short-Form General Health Survey. The instrument covers physical, role and social functioning, mental health, self-assessed health and physical pain. All variables were measured on a scale from zero to one hundred. The mental health variable includes five items concerning "general mood or affect, including depression, anxiety and positive well-being during the past month". It is thus the variable that most closely measures the psychological impact of illness. With the exception of the hypertensive, the chronically ill scored significantly poorer on all dimensions than the non-chronically ill. Interestingly, however, the differences in mean scores were much smaller on the mood dimension ("mental health") than on the other dimensions (typically 3-4 percentage points versus 10 to 15 percentage points).

In an explorative study, Selai and Rosser (1995) obtained quality of life ratings on a visual analogue scale running from zero to one hundred from 23 severely ill inpatients in a London hospital. The scores ranged from 30 to 100, with a mean of 64. By comparison, previous hypothetical valuations in a general population sample by means of the same visual analogue scale predicted a mean score in the order of 55 (authors' calculation based on Williams, 1995).

In a number of studies, convenience samples of healthy people and/or patients have been asked to value health states other than their own by means of the time trade-off technique (Torrance, 1986). The following are some examples of scores that have been elicited prior to the work of the EuroQol Group: walking stick: 0.78; walking frame: 0.58 (Bombardier *et al*, 1982); moderate angina: 0.83; severe angina: 0.53 (Read *et al*, 1984); removed breast, unconcerned: 0.80 (Richardson *et al*, 1989); removed breast, occasionally concerned: 0.70 (Buxton *et al*, 1987). These results may be compared with results from studies in which patients have been asked to evaluate their own health state by means of the time trade-off technique:

Churchill *et al* (1984) used the technique to measure quality of life in renal patients, of whom 42 were on haemodialysis, 17 on ambulant peritoneal dialysis, and 14 had transplants. The variability in willingness to sacrifice longevity to become well was striking, particularly in the haemodialysis group where there was an almost rectangular distribution ranging from 10 to 100 percent. The mean utility score in this group was 0.54.

Fryback *et al* (1993) studied health-related quality of life in a random sample of 1356 adults in a community population, using, among other instruments, a time trade-off questionnaire. Their report includes 25 chronic conditions that affected a sufficient number of people to allow calculations of mean TTO-scores with 95% confidence intervals less than 15 percentage points. The willingness to sacrifice longevity (WTSL) in order to be cured of one specific illness was not observed directly, as the TTO refers to becoming healthy and most subjects had more than one condition. However, the authors estimated that the conditions associated with the highest disutilities were insulin dependent diabetes (WTSL=24%), depression (17%), asthma (16%), and chronic bronchitis (14%). The willingness to sacrifice was only 5-8% in people with arthritis, severe back pain, migraine, angina, cataract, ulcer, colitis and sleep disorder.

Tsevat *et al* (1995) applied the time trade-off technique in 1438 seriously ill patients with a projected overall 6-month mortality rate of 50%. The patients had at least one of the following nine diseases: acute respiratory failure, acute exacerbation of severe chronic obstructive pulmonary disease, acute exacerbation of severe chronic congestive heart failure, chronic liver failure with cirrhosis, non-traumatic coma, colon cancer metastatic to the liver, metastatic non-small-cell carcinoma of the lung, multi-organ system failure with malignancy, and multi-organ system failure with sepsis. The subjects were asked to choose (hypothetically) between one year in the current state and a shorter time period as healthy. Responses varied widely. Mean willingness to sacrifice time was 27%, corresponding to a utility score of 0.73. 35% of the patients were unwilling to exchange any time in their current state for a shorter life in excellent health.

In a number of studies, patients' personal judgements of their own health and quality of life have been compared directly with judgements elicited from relatives and/or health care personnel (Nord, 1992). Some find a tendency for patients to score themselves higher than do relatives and health care personnel (Yager and Linn, 1981; Spitzer *et al*, 1981; Rubinstein *et al*, 1984; Magaziner *et al*, 1988; Pearlman and Uhlmann, 1988; Epstein *et al*, 1989; Rothman *et al*, 1991), while others find no systematic differences (Derogatis *et al*, 1976; Churchill *et al*, 1984; McCusker and Stoddard, 1984; Clipp and Elder, 1987; O'Brien and Francis, 1988; Slevin *et al*, 1988). We are not aware of studies that have reported opposite results.

11
Inconsistency and health state valuations

Paul Dolan and Paul Kind

11.1 ABSTRACT

Comparison of scaling methods used to value health states sometimes rests upon an examination of aggregate scores. This analysis is usually undertaken once "inconsistent" respondents have been excluded from the data. However, it is important to have information on the extent to which respondents are logically consistent when valuing health states. The degree of inconsistency will depend on how the health states are described, how the questionnaire is administered and who the respondents are. This paper analyses the inconsistency rates from two studies in which valuations for EuroQol health states were elicited using a visual analogue scale. The studies differed in design and incorporated several different variants of the standard EuroQol questionnaire, thus providing an opportunity to examine the relative importance of the different factors that were thought to affect inconsistency rates. Our general conclusions are that inconsistency rates are higher for postal than for interviewer-based surveys, possibly due to response bias, and that inconsistency rates are positively related to age and negatively related to educational attainment.

11.2 INTRODUCTION

A central task in the field of health status measurement involves eliciting valuations for health states using one or more of a number of different scaling methods, for example category rating, magnitude estimation, equivalence of numbers, graphical rating scales (Torrance, 1986). Individuals generally hold differing views and opinions on a wide range of issues relating to their everyday experiences, so that it might be expected that valuations for health states derived from different respondents would naturally vary also. It is not surprising, then, that within any given method there may be significant variability across population subgroups (for a review of the literature see Froberg and Kane, 1989). However, different scales of values have also been observed from the different scaling methods from the same respondents. There are many aspects of the measurement process which may be implicated in the diversity of results that are found in empirical studies, including the way in which health states are described (Boyd, 1982), the valuation method used (Read *et al*, 1984), and the characteristics of the respondent (Rosser and Kind, 1978).

It is perhaps useful to distinguish between "primary" inconsistencies that arise from intrinsic limitations of the human judgement process and "secondary" inconsistencies that result as a consequence of some aspect of the valuation procedure. Much of the

P. Kind et al. (eds.), EQ-5D concepts and methods, 139–146.

literature has focused on differences that arise as a result of these "secondary" inconsistencies, evidenced by researchers' emphasis on what Kahneman and Tversky refer to as "framing effects" (Kahneman and Tversky, 1981). The extent of inconsistencies due to "primary" factors is largely unknown. Much of the potential evidence on this matter is "lost" through the censoring of empirical data so that analysis is carried out only after respondents whose rankings fall to conform with *a priori* expectations have been excluded. This paper seeks to redress this imbalance and focuses on uncensored data. It reports on inconsistencies in health state valuations and looks at the factors which influence may them.

11.3 DATA

The analysis in this paper uses data from two studies undertaken as part of the Measurement and Valuation of Health Project conducted at the Centre for Health Economics at the University of York. Both studies incorporated a version of the EuroQol questionnaire (EuroQol Group, 1990). The first data set (LC) was obtained as part of a wider study of lay concepts of health, and utilised the original 6-dimensional form of the EuroQol classification. Self-completion questionnaires which record valuations for EuroQol health states were administered during face-to-face interviews conducted with young disabled adults and their carers, as well as with matched controls and a random sample from the community. The fieldwork was carried out in Dudley, Walsall and Wolverhampton during 1988. The second data set (F4) consisted of responses to a postal survey of patients registered with a large general practice in Frome, Somerset, and was carried out in 1991. The questionnaire was similar to that used in the LC study but utilised a revised 5-dimensional version of the EuroQol classification. The variants of this classification are shown in Table 11.1.

Table 11.1 The variants of the EuroQol questionnaire

	Questionaire variant					
Dimension	LC	F4A	F4B	F4C	F4D	F4E
Mobility	3	3	3	3	3	3
Self-Care	3	3	3	3	3	3
Work Activities	2					
Leisure Activities	2					
Usual Activities		3	3	3	3	3
Pain/Discomfort	3	3	3	3	3	3
Anxiety/Depression	2	3	3	3	3	3
Energy/Tiredness					2	2

The numbers in the boxes refer to the number of levels on each of the dimensions

All questionnaires asked respondents to describe their own health using the EuroQol descriptive system, and to rate their own health on a visual analogue scale (VAS) with 100 ('best imaginable health state') and 0 ('worst imaginable health state') as endpoints. Respondents then valued a standard set of 16 composite Euroqol states on a similar visual analogue scale. In addition, respondents were asked to record valuations for "death". Finally, respondents were asked a number of background questions relating to their age, sex, experience of illness and educational attainment. The two data sets present the opportunity to assess whether inconsistency rates are a function of:

(i) the mode of administration
(ii) the descriptive system used, and/or
(iii) the effect of different respondent characteristics.

11.4 DEFINING INCONSISTENCY

It can be assumed that discrete dimensions in both forms of the EuroQol descriptive systems constitute ordinal scales in which level i+1 < level i , for example having some problems with self-care (level 2) is worse than having no problem with self-care (level 1). Health states are formed by combining elements from each dimension and these composite descriptions may also be ordered according to their inherent ordinality. For any subset of such composite states it follows that there is an expected ordinal relationship between some, but not all pairs of states. For example, if state A is formed by combining levels 13221 respectively on each of the 5 (revised) dimensions, and state B is similarly formed by combining levels 12221, then it follows that state A is logically worse than state B, since for each dimension in state A the level is equal to or worse than the corresponding level for state B. For a respondent to meet perfectly the assumption of ordinality, the value they give to state A should be higher than the value given to state B when state B is 'logically' better on at least one dimension and no worse on the other dimensions.

Only some pairs of the EuroQol states used in the two surveys stand in a logically defined ordinal relationship. There are 83 such pairs possible for the LC data set, and 75 for the F4 data set. For each respondent it is possible to calculate the number of times an expected logically consistent ranking occurs, and hence to calculate an inconsistency rate (expressed as a percentage) using as the denominator the maximum possible number of such logical pairings. This statistic is comparable to the coefficient of inconsistency described by Kendall with regard to paired comparisons data (Kendall, 1962).

Each group of respondents in the LC data was analysed separately since the five sub-samples differed in respect of their background characteristics, not least in their experience of illness. The F4 study used five variants of the same questionnaire and since each questionnaire differed slightly, responses were not pooled.

11.5 RESULTS

Table 11.2 shows the mean and median inconsistency rates for each sub-sample in the two studies. First, median inconsistency rates are lower than mean inconsistency rates for all sub samples, particularly those in the F4 study. This suggests that a few respondents with very high inconsistency rates are biasing the mean upwards. In the F4 study, where the difference between the mean and the median is most marked, there are 31 respondents (ranging from 3 in questionnaire E to 9 in questionnaire D) who have inconsistency rates above 50%.

Table 11.2 Percentage inconsistency rates for the lay concepts and Frome IV studies

Lay Concepts	n	Mean	(S.D.)	Median	(IQR)
General Population	163	13.3	(9.3)	10.8	(8.4-14.5)
Disabled Group	81	11.6	(6.6)	9.6	(7.2-12.7)
Disabled Control	69	19.7 *	(16.6)	15.6 *	(9.6-11.1)
Carer Group	80	10.8	(4.7)	10.4	(8.4-14.2)
Carer Control	95	13.0	(6.7)	12.0	(8.4-16.9)

Frome IV	n	Mean	(S.D.)	Median	(IQR)
A	95	10.9	(19.9)	2.7	(1.3-9.3)
B	96	8.6	(17.1)	2.7	(0-9.3)
C	96	9.8	(19.1)	2.7	(0-7.7)
D	80	9.8	(17.2)	2.7	(1.3-10.3)
E	95	6.7	(12.3)	2.7	(0-6.7)

* Significantly different from other groups ($p < 0.01$)

An analysis of these respondents showed that 18 had responses that were clustered around the two endpoints of the scale. This finding may indicate a misinterpretation of the labels 'best imaginable health state' and 'worst imaginable health state' since it is possible that these 18 respondents thought they were to locate the states on the scale according to how well they could imagine being in them (van Busschbach, 1994). This would explain why states which could be the considered to be the most difficult to imagine - dead and unconscious - were either unvalued or given a score of 0 by all of these respondents. In contrast, there are only 4 respondents in the LC study (all of them in the disabled group of respondents) who appear to be interpreting the instructions in this way.

Second, the median inconsistency rates for the LC sub-samples are significantly higher than those for the F4 sub-samples[1]. In addition, the modal inconsistency rate for the LC sub-samples is around 10%, whilst for F4 it is 0% in 3 of the 5 sub-samples, and below 3% in the other two. These differences suggest that the 6-D descriptive system used in the LC study may be more prone to rankings that violate the logical ordering than the revised 5-D one. However, two of the F4 questionnaire variants contained an extra dimension effectively making these 6-D descriptive systems too, and there were no differences in the inconsistency rates of respondents to these questionnaires compared to the others in F4. Therefore, differences in the median inconsistency rates observed appear to be explained by factors other than the descriptive system alone.

These differences in inconsistency rates between LC and F4 might be explained in terms of the different ways in which the LC and F4 studies were conducted, the former being interview-based and the latter being a postal survey. In the F4 study, if potential respondents, for whatever reasons, experienced difficulties with the questionnaire, they were not obliged to reply. In addition, no reminders were sent out after the original mailing. Thus, there must be an inevitable response bias with those returning their questionnaires being a self-selected group of respondents who understood (or at least thought they understood) the questionnaire. Of course, there is the possibility of response bias to interview-based studies such as LC but there would seem to be less scope for refusal under such circumstances.

Third, the disabled control group of respondents in the LC study (i.e. young, fit people who may not care or think much about illness) had higher inconsistency rates than the other groups, particularly the disabled group. This suggests that those with experience of illness may be less inconsistent than those with no such experience. However, when respondents were categorised according to their current and past illness experience, Mann-Whitney U tests revealed no significant differences, suggesting that experience of illness is not closely linked to inconsistency rates.

11.6 THE INFLUENCE OF OTHER SOCIO-DEMOGRAPHIC FACTORS

In both studies, there were no significant differences in inconsistency rates according to the sex or the smoking behaviour of the respondent. When inconsistency rates are analysed according to age group, however, different patterns emerge from the two studies, as is shown in Table 11.3. For the general population[2] sub-sample of LC there is no significant difference between the younger (16-35 inclusive) and older (56 and over) respondents in terms of their inconsistency rates. With F4, however, older

1. Throughout this paper significance is reported at the 1% level.
2. It was only possible to analyse the random population sample of the Lay Concepts data since the carer and carer control groups contained too few "young" respondents and the disabled and disabled control groups contained too few "old" respondents.

respondents in every sub-sample have significantly higher levels of inconsistency. This finding is intuitively appealing since with increasing age, physical and intellectual capacities may deteriorate, with a presumed tendency to increased logically inconsistent responses.

Table 11.3 The effect of age on inconsistency rates

	n1	n2	n3	Median 1	(IQR)	Median 2	(IOR)	Median 3	(IQR)
Lay Concepts									
General Population	73	54	34	9.6	(8.4-12.7)	10.8	(8.1-14.0)	12.0	(8.1-17.5)
Frome IV									
A	28	35	31	2.7	(1.3-8.0)	1.3	(0-5.3)	6.7	(1.3-30.7)
B	24	41	31	2.7	(0.3-9.0)	1.3	(0-5.3)	6.7	(1.3-16.0)
C	27	43	26	1.3	(0-6.7)	2.7	(0-8.0)	2.7	(0-37.7)
D	21	36	22	1.3	(0.7-14.0)	2.7	(1.3-9.0)	4.0	(0-13.3)
E	21	42	32	2.7	(1.3-6.7)	1.3	(0-5.3)	4.7	(1.3-10.0)

Group 1 = those aged 16-35

Group 2 = those aged 36-55

Group 3 = those aged 56+

Table 11.4 presents inconsistency rates for those with and without further education. Again the results from all F4 sub-samples are intuitively appealing since those with lower levels of education, and therefore perhaps lower levels of literacy or ability to interpret the composite health states, have higher levels of inconsistency. The LC data follows a similar pattern but, although median inconsistency rates are higher for the less educated in every sub-sample, this difference is not significant at the 1% level.

Table 11.4 The effect of education on inconsistency rates

	n1	n2	Median 1	(IQR)	Median 2	(IQR)
Lay Concepts						
General Population	78	85	10.2	(7.2-14.5)	12.0	(8.4-15.7)
Disabled Group	22	59	9.6	(7.2-12.3)	9.6	(7.2-13.3)
Disabled Control	50	18	14.5	(9.3-18.7)	18.1	(13.0-15.9)
Carer Group	61	19	9.6	(7.2-12.0)	14.5	(10.8-15.6)
Carer Control	25	70	9.6	(6.0-14.5)	2.7	(9.6-6.9)
Frome IV						
A	58	37	2.3	(1.3-8.0)	5.3	(0.7-12.0)
B	48	48	2.3	(1.3-5.3)	4.0	(0-13.3)
C	53	43	1.3	(0-5.3)	4.0	(1.3-30.7)
D	38	41	2.7	(1.0-8.0)	4.0	(1.3-11.3)
E	50	68	1.3	(0-5.3)	4.0	(1.3-8.7)

n1 = those with further training

n2 = those with minimum education

11.7 DISCUSSION

Overall, the inconsistency rates associated with using the visual analogue scale to value EuroQol health states are encouraging. Median inconsistency rates of around 10% were obtained from the LC study whilst every sub-sample of the F4 study produced rates below 3%. Of those respondents with high inconsistency rates, it is possible that some may have misinterpreted the terms 'best imaginable health state' and 'worst imaginable health state'.

Perhaps the most important finding is that inconsistency rates are lower for postal as compared to interviewer-based questionnaires. The "self-selecting" nature of respondents to postal questionnaires was posited as one possible explanation of this. It seems quite plausible that the motivation, attention to detail, and level of performance of respondents may be influenced by the settings in which they complete the questionnaire.

With respect to the factors influencing inconsistency, it appears that rates are positively related to age and negatively related to educational attainment. These results confirm *a priori* expectations. A recent study which used the same visual analogue scale reported higher inconsistency rates for those with a low self-rated health status and those with personal past experience of illness (Kind *et al*, 1993). Such results were not reproduced in this study although it should be noted that the Kind *et al* study examined inconsistency rates in valuations based on a different health state descriptive system. This may suggest that inconsistency may be more a function of the descriptive system than the valuation technique.

The lowest median level of inconsistency recorded was about 3% which suggests that an intrinsic residual inconsistency of this order could be anticipated in any study using a visual analogue scale to elicit health state valuations. The lack of unambiguous results leaves open the question of the origin of this inconsistency. It seems likely to be determined by both "primary" and "secondary" factors but the balance between the two remains indeterminate.

This paper addresses an issue that has been largely ignored by researchers in the health state measurement field. "Inconsistent" respondents have been reported in other studies but often only as a justification for their exclusion from subsequent analysis. Only by looking more closely at these respondents and analysing why inconsistencies occur in the first place will our understanding of health status measurement be enhanced. This paper has provided a framework in which other studies can report inconsistency, and provides a benchmark against which inconsistency rates can be compared.

Presented at the EuroQol Plenary Meeting: Rotterdam, The Netherlands, 1993

11.8 REFERENCES

Boyd N F, Sutherland N J, Ciampi A, Tibshirani R, Till J E, Harwood A. A comparison of methods of assessing voice quality in laryngeal cancer. In: Choices in health care: decision making and evaluation of effectiveness. Department of Health Administration, University of Toronto, 1982.

Busschbach J, Hessing D J, Charro, F T de. Observations on 100 students filling in the EuroQol questionnaire. Quality of Life Research 1994:3(1):71-72.

EuroQol Group. EuroQol - a new facility for the measurement of health-related quality of life. Health Policy 1990;16:199-208.

Froberg D G, Kane R L. Methodology for measuring health state preferences III: population and context effects. Journal of Clinical Epidemiology 1989;42:585-92.

Kahneman D, Tversky A. The framing of decisions and the psychology of choice. The framing of decisions and the psychology of choice. Science 1981;211(4481):453-458.

Kendall M G. Rank correlation methods. 3rd edition, London: Griffin, 1962:146.

Kind P, Dolan P, Gudex C M, Williams A H. Inconsistency and the judgment of health state valuation: a comparison of three scaling methods. IRSS workshop October 1992. University of York.

Read J L, Quinn R J, Berwick DM, Fineberg H V, Weinstein MC. Preferences for health outcomes: comparison of assessment methods, Medical Decision Making 1984;4:315-329.

Rosser R, Kind P. A scale of valuations of states of illness: is there a social consensus? International Journal of Epidemiology 1978;7:347-358.

Torrance G W. Measurement of health state utilities for economic appraisal. Journal of Health Economics 1986;5:1-30.

12
Issues in the harmonisation of valuation and modeling

Paul Krabbe, Frank de Charro and Marie-Louise Essink-Bot

12.1 INTRODUCTION

For the last two years modeling has been at the top of the agenda of the EuroQol Group. In particular, due to the major research task performed by the York Group (MVH project) progress has been made in developing and specifying a statistical model. Such a model is urgently required for estimating all the 243 health states of the EuroQol descriptive system.

Based on the "valuations" of 45 EuroQol health states obtained from a sample of English inhabitants, a model could be developed. This model needed to be precise and valid enough to estimate valuations for the 198 EuroQol health states which were not valued in the study. The estimates for all the 243 EuroQol health states were termed as the "tariff". Elicitation of the 45 health state descriptions was accomplished using two different methods: visual analogue scaling (VAS) and the time trade-off (TTO) method.

We have great admiration for the major task the York Group has undertaken. This contribution has led the EuroQol Group close to its initial goal: a numeric index for a range of health states suitable to incorporate in medical decisions and to serve as an instrument for health policymakers. On the other hand, the modeling efforts of the York Group have raised a number of questions concerning the procedure to elicit values, transformations of the data, and the model itself. Many of the questions mentioned in this paper not only apply to the York study but are also issues that are discussed in the scientific field as a whole.

The purpose of this paper is to highlight some of the prominent questions and related problems associated with valuation and modeling in relation to the modeling study of the York Group.

12.2 MAJOR DECISION POINTS IN THE PROCESS OF VALUATION AND MODELING

Aggregation or individual values

One of the most basic decisions that can be made in the process of modeling the EuroQol tariff is whether to model on the individual valuations or on the group outcomes. When using group outcomes individual information is lost. On the other

P. Kind et al. (eds.), EQ-5D concepts and methods, 147–156.

hand, if the purpose is to eliminate extreme individual valuations, aggregation may be helpful for further computations.

Normalisation of the data: skewness and kurtosis

Subjects valuing EuroQol health states are forced to value between 0 and 100 when valuation takes place, whether using the EuroQol Instrument or trade-off methods such as standard gamble (SG) and TTO. Non-normal distribution of valuations of health states will occur for the very good and the very bad health states. For very good health states (e.g. "12111", "11121") most of these valuations are close to 100. The "barriers" of the valuation scale are forcing the distribution of health states with mean values close to 0 or 100, to non-normal distributions of the scores.

Non-normal distributions can be corrected by performing transformations on the data. Logit-transformations and arcsine-transformations often give good results. Transformation must take place before modeling. Backward transformation must be performed after the most suitable model is selected and the "tariff" is estimated. So, estimated health states by a model based on transformed valuations will finally be represented within the same range as the original valuations.

Specifying the model: dummies

modeling within the regression model is adequate for the type of data gathered in valuations of health states. Since for the independent (predictor) variables we are not dealing with continuous data (e.g. age, income) but with ordinal data (level 1,2 or 3), dummy variables have to be constructed. A complicating factor is that different forms of coding are available. The one most frequently used is called dummy coding. However, it is possible to use one of the other two forms of coding: effect coding and orthogonal coding. Each type of coding has its own features and consequences.

When interactions have to be part of the model, the whole exercise will be much more complicated. In this case the design of the study requires a specified selection of the 243 health states to be able to estimate all first-order interaction effects.

Methods: the consequence of using a specific elicitation method

Each of the established methods that are used for the elicitation of valuations of health states has its own drawbacks and complicating aspects. For instance the SG method is difficult to understand for people and is susceptible to "risk-aversion". The TTO method, although easier to comprehend, has to deal with "time preference". This latter factor consists of two intertwined sub-factors: a discounting effect and a sequence effect. Valuations made by the VAS method are not gathered under a trade-off task.

The position of dead

In both SG and TTO the state of "dead" occupies a specific position. In Torrance's original operationalization of TTO, "dead" follows the shorter period in perfect health. Normally, when a health state is valued as worse than "dead" (indicated by a preference to die immediately instead of living any number of years in the state to be valued) a modification for the TTO (and SG) method is necessary. For the valuation of EuroQol health states this should be, for TTO, the replacement of "dead" with the description of the EuroQol health state valued worse than "dead" and the replacement of the stationary health state (normally the state to be valued) with "dead". Since "perfect health" (here "11111") is set to 1 and dead is set equal to zero - which is the convention in utility measurement - health states worse than dead will be valued negatively. The lower bound for these negatively valued health states is not -1, but depends on the interval of the number of years in the TTO exercise.

If "dead" had been the label of the lowest endpoint of the EuroQol-VAS, a two-stage procedure for the valuation of states worse-than-dead would also have been necessary with this method. However, for theoretical and practical reasons the EuroQol Group has chosen 'worst imaginable health state' to label the low endpoint, and a separate rating of dead.

12.3 THE YORK STUDY

Individual versus group outcomes

In the York study modeling took place on individual valuations and on aggregated data. In order to make comparisons between modeling on the means and modeling on the medians, to examine the effect of eliminating extreme individual valuations, both types of modeling should preferably take place on aggregated data. It seems that the York Group has modelled with "means" based on an individual level and with medians based on a group level. The question here is whether the effect of the measure of central tendency (mean *versus* median) could be better studied if both measures of central tendency were based at the group level.

Normalisation data

No comments on the issue of this type of transformation of the data before modeling, with backward transformations afterwards, could be found by us in the papers of the York Group.

Data transformations: complete and partial

Both the VAS and TTO data of the York study were transformed. After transformation VAS and TTO data had an upper bound of 1 and a lower bound of -1.

VAS: VAS data was transformed so that full health equals 1 and dead equals 0 after transformation. In particular the transformation of the VAS data, performed on the individual responses, may lead to complications for the modeling. By forcing the valuation of dead to zero, the standard deviation for the health state dead becomes zero too. On the other hand, variation centred around the other health states is artificially modified, which may have major implications for the estimation of models. In particular the worse health states valued in the same region as dead are artificially loaded with additional variations.

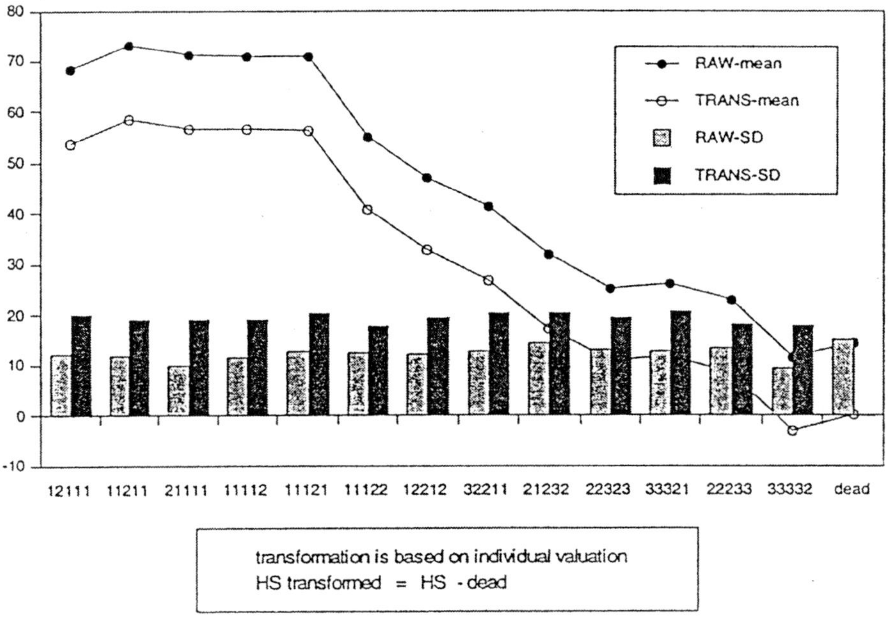

Figure 12.1 Testing the effect of forcing dead to zero (complete transformation) for the VAS method on the data of the HESTEM experiments (Rotterdam)

It should be noted that dead is the "health state" most valued inaccurately because of the lack of agreement among respondents, and because valuing a non-health state such as dead is more or less a metaphysical exercise. The variation for dead is therefore high. When forcing dead to become zero, this variability will be transferred to all the other health states (see Figure 12.1).

TTO: This trade-off method yields values that express the number of years that people are willing to give up to stay in the health state to be valued. In the York study a standard time period (t) of 10 years was used and time periods could be expressed in steps of 1/4 years. The total time period (10) minus the number of years people are willing to give up (v), divided by the total time period (10) are called utilities (u; see Equation 12.1). These utilities express the valuation of a specific health state on a range from zero (health state equal preferred to dead) to 1 (perfect health).

$$u = \frac{t - v}{t} \Rightarrow \frac{10 - v}{10} \tag{12.1}$$

For health states that are valued worse than dead the TTO task is a modified one (see under: "the position of dead") and the equation for computing utilities becomes:

$$u = \frac{v / t}{1 - (v / t)} \Rightarrow \frac{v / 10}{1 - (v / 10)} \tag{12.2}$$

The range of utilities that can be elicited for health states worse than dead is not simply a mirror image of the utility range of the better-than-dead health states. Worse-than-dead utilities range from 0 to a minimum number that depends on the number of steps used for the TTO method. In the York study these steps of 1/4 years in a total time period of 10 years gives 40 possible valuation categories. In Table 12.1 an overview is presented with a selection of initial trade-off values for health states valued better than dead and valued worse than dead.

The specific nature of equation (12.2) can best be demonstrated for a health state that is valued with a trade-off value of -5 (see: Table 12.1 and Figure 12.2).

Table 12.1 The trade-offs, computed utilities (computation different for health states valued worse than dead than for those health states which are valued better than dead) and the values after the York transformation for the TTO method

		Trade-offs	Utilities	Partial transformation (transformed utilities)
Health states worse than dead	'Worst imaginable health state'	-9.75	-39	-0.975
		-9.5	-19	-0.95
		8	4	0.8
		-7	-2.33	-0.7
		-6	-1.5	-0.6
		-5	-1	-0.5
		-4	-0.66	-0.4
		-3	-0.43	-0.3
		-2	-0.25	-0.2
	Worse than dead	-1	-0.11	-0.1
	Health state equal to death	0	0	0
Health states better than dead	Worst health state	1	0.1	0.1
		2	0.2	0.2
		3	0.3	0.3
		4	0.4	0.4
		5	0.5	0.5
		6	0.6	0.6
		7	0.7	0.7
		8	0.8	0.8
		9	0.9	0.9
	Best imaginable health state	10	1	1

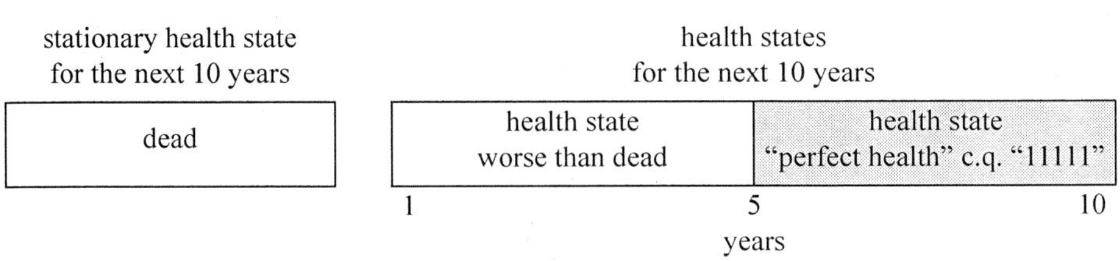

Figure 12.2 Example of the situation for the time trade-off elicitation method of valuing a worse-than-dead health state two times worse (trade-off value = -5 years; utility = -1) than the (non) health state 'dead'

We think that to overcome the extreme negative values (utilities) and to obtain a scale with an equal range from zero (dead) to minus 1 the TTO data was partially backward transformed by the York Group using the following equation:

$$if\ u < 0\ then: u_t = \frac{u}{1-u}; u = utility, u_t = transformed\ utility \qquad (12.3)$$

So for the minimum score under the condition that a health state is valued worse than dead (-39 in the York study) the transformed value becomes:

$$\frac{u}{1-u} \Rightarrow \frac{-39}{1-(-39)} = -0.975 \qquad (12.4)$$

This partial transformation for the health states valued worse than dead has led to discussion about the consequences and implications of this uncommon transformation.

Formally, utilities express the real position of valuations of health states in relation to the fixed positions of "perfect health" (1) and "dead" (0). The most extreme valuation that could be elicited within the MVH-project was -39. This value implies that health states with such a negative valuation are indeed valued at 39 times worse than the (health) state dead itself. This consequence has nothing to do with the strategy of the York Group but everything to do with utility theory and the underlying concepts common in the scientific field of decision-makers and economists. Whether or not this assumption is correct is a totally different question, although of the highest importance if we are to overcome the mystification concearning the issue of health states worse-than-dead.

Another phenomenon related to the use of negative values for worse-than-dead health states (no matter whether we use the utilities: 0 ... -39; or the partial transformed data: 0 ... -1) is that in QALY-calculations negative values of health states may result in complicated computations. In particular policymakers may have strong objections working with negative values.

It can be seen in Table 12.1 that the partial transformation for all utilities below zero produces the same proportional values as the initial trade-off values. The advantage in the two computational steps (Equations 12.1, 12.2 and 12.3) is thus not clear to us.

Note that the type of transformations that were performed by the York Group are contrary to the type of transformation normally mentioned, namely the class of transformations discussed in this paper under "normalization".

Figure 12.3 shows the dramatic effect of backward transformation, when negative values are transformed for the TTO method by equation (12.4).

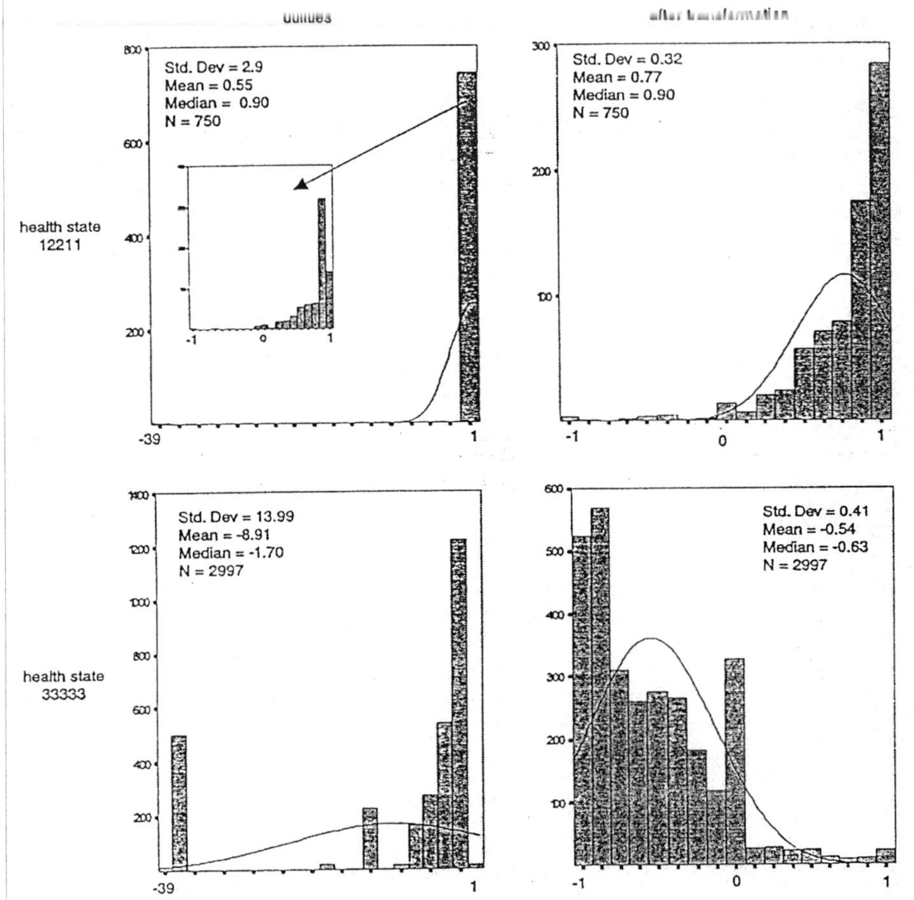

Figure 12.3 The effect on the distribution of backward transformation for valuations valued worse than dead by the time trade-off method

Towards the Dolan-N3 model

One of the elegant characteristics of the Dolan-N3 model is that the modeling has been performed under the random effects (RE) model. The model has been specified with parsimony (i.e., simplicity) of the model as an important criterion. However, the specification of the dependent variables (dummies) and especially the introduction of the N3 dummy (which indicates that any dimension of the valued health state has level 3) have led to some discussion.

For the Dolan-N3 model five basic dummies (MO, SC, UA, PD, AD) were constructed for each EuroQol dimension: 0 if level = 1, 1 if level = 2, and 2 if level = 3. Formally these are not dummies but normal continuous dependent variables. The effect of the move from level 1 to level 2 is therefore expected to be the same as the effect from level 2 to level 3.

Five additional dummies (M2, S2, U2, P2, A2) were incorporated in the model, indicating for each EuroQol dimension if level 3 is actual or not (dummies specified as: 0 if level is 1 or 2, 1 if level is 3). These five dummies are part of the model to overcome the fixed effects that were introduced by the first set of "dummies". The question here is: why not use the standard solution for dummy specification? Thus, for each dimension two dummies could be employed, namely dummy A: 0 if level is not 1, 1 if level is 1; and dummy B: 0 if level is not 3, 1 if level is 3.

Finally the introduction of the N3-dummy may introduce redundancy, because each level 3 for all the five EuroQol dimensions is already specified by the 10 other dummies.

12.4 ALTERNATIVE STRATEGIES

Aggregation or not

Although the use of medians (implying aggregation of the data) has the advantage that the influence of extreme individual valuations is strongly reduced, modeling on all the information and, therefore, on individual valuations has unarguable benefits. These include: being able to use special models (for example: the RE model), the possibility to detect groups with different response patterns; controlling for background variables; solid modeling practice; and so forth. Non-normal distribution of valuations of health states and the influence of extreme valuations should preferably be overcome and eliminated by customary transformation of the data, inclusion criteria, and other strategies. The use of the TTO method with the valuation of severe health states (if valued worse than dead) may yield to extreme negative valuations. It is for this reason that the York Group has also produced tariffs based on median values.

How to overcome being tangled up in transformations

An alternative strategy to the one performed by the York Group would be the selection of 'worst imaginable health state' instead of dead as the fixed reference state for 0 (zero). In conventional TTO (and SG), "dead" only serves as a benchmark. "Dead" is not an essential part of either method, nor is the use of perfect health at the other extreme. Logically any two pairs of reference states are suitable as long as they "embrace" the state to be valued and their utility value is known. The TTO procedure should allow for the use of reference states other than those used conventionally. Furthermore, it is a matter of taste or convention to anchor the value of "dead" at 0 (zero). Inevitably this convention leads to the assigning of negative values ot the worst health states, regardless of the health description system used.

Finally, we wish to be able to compare SG and TTO data with standard EuroQol VAS-data. In the EuroQol standard questionnaire "dead" is rated in a separate valuation task. With the additional measurement of the value for "dead", scores on the "healthy-worst imaginable health state" scale can be transformed to a 0-1 perfect healthy-dead scale of values.

modeling revisited?

Several questions have been raised in the wake of the extensive modeling exercises of the York Group and others. Some aspects that may be worthwhile for further discussion and research are mentioned below:

(i) The use of health state "33333" as a reference health state instead of the non-health state "dead" for VAS and TTO.
(ii) Normalisation of the data to overcome the non-normal dispersion of some of the valued health states.
(iii) Using VAS values instead of TTO values (utilities) to overcome time-preference effects.
(iv) Testing the effects of the different dummy strategies.
(v) Simplifying the specifications of the regression model.
(vi) Incorporation of first-order interaction effects in the model.

Presented at the EuroQol Plenary Meeting: Barcelona, Spain, 1995

13
Estimating a parametric relation between health description and health valuation using the EuroQol Instrument

Ben van Hout and Joseph McDonnell

13.1 INTRODUCTION

Although the word QALY may be permitted during a game of Scrabble between health economists there is still a long way to go before consensus is reached about its meaning and its usefulness. There are still a number of methodological and practical questions to be answered, too many to handle In one research project. This, among others, is one of the raisons d'existence of the EuroQol Group. a network of European researchers who are trying to develop a common methodology regarding the valuation of various health states. As part of the work carried out by this Group, we will address one of the practical questions, namely the estimation of a parametric relationship between health descriptions and the value attained to these descriptions.

One of the methodological starting points of the EuroQol Group is the assumption that health is a multidimensional concept which can be characterised by a description of scores on five dimensions. These dimensions are:

1 Mobility
2 Self-care
3 Usual activities
4 Pain/discomfort
5 Anxiety/depression.

Within the defined concept every individual health state can be described by using a vector X (X_1,X_2,...,X_5) in which X represents each dimension. We will presume that each dimension is essentially continuous and that it can take values between some fixed end points [a,b], for example [1,3]. Then, each health state may be characterised as a point x (x1,x2,...x5) in a five-dimensional space. The EuroQol Group has chosen a common core of three descriptors per dimension: two which mark the limits of its space, a good one and a bad one, and one which lies between these. With five dimensions and three descriptors per dimension, there are $3^5 = 243$ descriptions of health states which can be described in numbers. The description [1,1,1,1,1] represents the best and the description [3,3,3,3,3] corresponds to the worst health state.

Most commonly the EuroQol Group uses postal questionnaires by which respondents are asked to assign values to a number of selected heafth states. All health states are valued using a thermometer with at the top the description 'best imaginable health

P. Kind et al. (eds.), EQ-5D concepts and methods, 157–170.

state' and at the bottom 'worst imaginable health state'. Only a limited number of health states can be assigned values in this way. Although some of the possible health states might never occur, some will, and may never be valued in a questionnaire. Therefore, we think it is useful to explore the possibilities of developing a parametric model on the basis of which expectations might be formulated about values for all possible health states. In algebraic terms we are searching for the following relation:

$$V = V(X,\alpha) \tag{13.1}$$

in which V measures the valuation of the heath state described by the vector X and in which α is a vector of parameters.

The problems that will be explored here may be illustrated after considering the structure of the available data. These consist of the answers to N-questionnaires in which K health states have been valued by samples of the general population. Assuming that every respondent differs, the observations can be represented as follows:

$$u_{ij} = u_{ij}(x_i, \alpha_j) + e_{ij} \qquad i = 1 \ldots K \qquad j = 1 \ldots N \tag{13.2}$$

Here u_{ij} is the value that respondent j has assigned to health state i; $u_{ij}(x_i, \alpha_j)$ is the functional form of the individual's value function and e_{ij} measures the difference between the observed value arid the predicted value. As an analogue to linear regression the e_{ij} represent measurement errors and the effects of mis-specification. The core of our research concentrates on three problems. First, we have to identify the criterium that will be used to estimate the parameters (mostly based on the e_{ij}). Second, we have to identity the characteristics of the scales of u and x. Finally we have to identify the model. We will treat these problems separately.

13.2 THE IDENTIFICATION OF A CRITERIUM FUNCTION

The choice of the criterium function may depend on the point of view from which we look at our data. We distinguish between an individual and a societal point of view.

From the individual point of view we may analyse every dataset from each individual separately and we may estimate various functional forms with their corresponding parameters. Different criteria can be used to estimate the parameters. The most natural option is the minimization of the differences between the observed and predicted valuations choosing various metrics. We should realise, however, that there are several alternatives. One alternative might be the minimization of the differences between the orderings between all subsequent points.

Estimation from the societal point of view means that we must try to find a model which represents the value that society asslgns to the different health states. We have to find:

$$u^*_j = u^*(x_j, \alpha) + e_j \tag{13.3}$$

Our observations give only information about individual values and so we have to find some aggregation procedure to estimate u^*_j. In doing this, we have to realise that we are not only minimizing measurement errors and unobserved heterogeneity, but are also trying to maximise consensus between individuals. Again, we may follow at least two procedures.

The first procedure may be to calculate the u^*_j from the individual u_{ij}. For this purpose we may use the mean, the mode or the median value. Using averages might be regarded as a utilitarian procedure while using the median or mode might be regarded as being based on a voting principle. Having made a choice about the general tendency measure, the procedure is analogous to the procedure from the individual point of view. We have to choose a criterium function and again we may choose between various options.

The second procedure may be to use the individual observations directly by assuming that;

$$u_{ij} = u^*(x_j, \alpha) + e_{ij} \tag{13.4}$$

and find the societal value function by an appropriate choice of the criterium function.

In this paper, we have limited ourselves to the options from the societal point of view using the Euclidean metric, minimizing the sum of squared residuals. The main reason for this choice is of course that it is very easy to use and that the resutts can easily be interpreted. On methodological grounds, however, other criteria might be preferred. Choosing other criterium functions will certainly be a topic for further research.

13.3 THE SCALE

The relationship that we are trying to estimate concerns, on the one hand, values on a scale with unknown properties and on the other hand descriptors of health dimensions measured on scales with similar unknown properties. Consequently, we will have to make some assumptions.

We emphasize that we will not address the question of the meaning of the values assigned to the descriptions. Whether this measures utility or something else is not of concern here. It does not affect our problem. About the property of the scale we will assume that it is an interval scale on the individual level. This means that the difference between 0.2 and 0.4 is equal to the difference between 0.4 and 0.8 for each individual.

The question to what extent we may compare a difference of 0.2 and 0.4 for one individual to another may be interpreted not only as a question concerning scaling but also of aggregation. Both problems are related to each other. As mentioned before we may, as an alternative to taking the central tendency measures, use the individual observations as the starting point for our estimations. Minimizing least squares without restrictions on the parameters would result in parameter estimates that are identical to the results on the basis of the average values. This is not necessarily true when we rescale the observations of each individual assigning the value 0 to point [33333] and the value 1 to point [11111] which - in our opinion - is an interesting exercise from a methodological point of view. By doing this we normalise each persons' scale on a [0,1] scale and disregard the differences between [11111] and the so called 'best imaginable health state' and between [33333] and the 'worst imaginable health state'. These differences may not be a reflection of differences in people's values but may reflect their visions about potential health states between these extreme points.

The second problem regarding scaling concerns the scale of the dimensions. The EuroQol Group has identified three points per dimension. Two points represent the borders of each dimension describing a very good and a very bad possibility. The third descriptor concerns a state somewhere in the middle. We may quantify these scales by choosing an arbitrary range [a,b]. While the choice of a and b does not matter, the choice of the mid-point does. We may choose a value in the middle $((a+b)/2)$ or we may try to estimate this value. The difference between both options is related to the choice of the model. In the next section we return to this subject.

13.4 THE MODEL

There are at least two assumptions that can be made about the functional relationship between the dimensions and our value function. First, we assume the preference function to be continuous and twice differentiable in its arguments, and second we assume first order derivates to be positive. The first assumption means that we believe that an infinitely small change in each dimension leads to an infinitely small change in the value attained to the health state. The second assumption means that we assume that a better score on each dimension leads to a higher valuation of the corresponding health state. Although both assumptions may sound plausible we should realize that they both may be violated by health states such as 'unconscious'. Having made our assumptions there are a number of different functional forms to consider.

For practical reasons, we will only consider two, an additive form and a multiplicative form. The additive form is written as:

$$u(x) = \alpha_0 + \sum_{i=1}^{5} \alpha_i u_i(x_i) \tag{13.5}$$

The multiplicative form, in which account is taken of first order multiplicative effects, is written as:

$$u(x) = \alpha_0 + \sum_{i=1}^{5} \alpha_i u_i(x_i) + \sum_{i=1}^{5} \sum_{j=i+1}^{5} \alpha_{ij} u_i(x_i) u_j(x_j) \tag{13.6}$$

A model in which account is also taken of second order interactions, but in a restricted way, is the following, which was used earlier by Torrance *et al*, 1982:

$$u(\alpha) = \left(\frac{1}{\alpha}\right)\left[\prod_{i=1}^{5} \{1 + \alpha\alpha_i u_i(x_i)\} - 1\right] \tag{13.7}$$

In all equations we see $u_i(x_i)$ instead of x_i representing the possibility that the effect of each dimension enters the functional form in a non-linear way. A problem which is not confined to the EuroQol Instrument concerns the identification of the partial value functions $u_i(x_i)$. As we are not certain about whether our mid-point takes the value 0.5, for example, we may not be able to identify the non-linear function $u_i(x_i)$, Let us assume, for example, that we have only one dimension and that the mid-point v(0.5) is scored at a value 0.7. This may be interpreted as a non-linearity, but the same observation can be explained by assuming a linear model and by assuming that the score 0.5, should be 0.7.

13.5 DATA

In the Rotterdam survey four different questionnaires were used. They differed from each other in the pages on which respondents were asked to some value health states using a thermometer offering values between 0 and 100. Four different pages each with 8 health states were discerned, namely A, A', B and B'. Version I contained the pages A and B, version II A' and B', version III A and B', and version IV contained the pages A' and B. Each page contained the best and the worst health states. Twenty four additional health states were defined, one of them being the state 'unconscious'. So, additionally 23 health states were evaluated.

Each questionnaire was sent to 350 households. Overall response was 70.3%. For our purposes we used a selection of the questionnaires. First, we only used completed questionnaires, Second, we disregarded all respondents who had given answers that were logically Inconsistent. if respondents gave higher or lower values to health states which were logically better or worse we disregarded all their values. For our estimates we used the following number of questionnaires:

Version I	115	Version II	98
Version III	93	Version IV	116

As a consequence, we had:
422 valuations of 11111 and 33333

208 valuations of page A (6 additional descriptions)
231 valuations of page B (5 additional descriptions)
214 valuations of page A' (6 additional descriptions)
191 valuations of page B' (6 additional descriptions).

13.6 RESULTS

On the basis of these data we have estimated linear and non-linear models taking various perspectives.. The first estimates concern the linear model and are based on our central tendency measures. Figure 13.1 presents the valuation of the various health states using the three general tendency measures: the average, the mode, and the median. They are sorted according to the average.

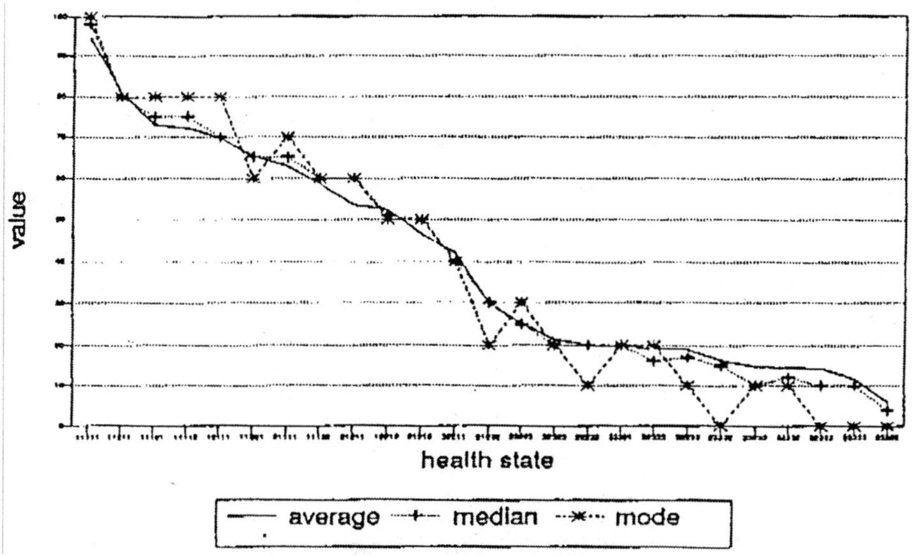

Figure 13.1 Health state values from the EuroQol Rotterdam survey

13.7 THE LINEAR MODEL

Table 13.1 presents estimates of the linear model without restrictions. The dimensions are scaled on a [0,1] scale, the best descriptors valued at 1, the worst at 0, and the mid-descriptors are valued at 0.5. The values are scaled on a [0,100] scale. The differences between the estimates for the various general tendency measures are substantial. While the estimates based on the average assign the highest weight to mobility, the estimates based on the mode assign the highest weight to usual activities. Standard errors are presented between parentheses but we should emphasize that the common interpretation is not correct as the errors are not normally distributed. In Table 13.2 we present estimates of the linear model in which dummy/variables are induded to be able to estimate the value of the mid-descriptors. Instead of standard errors we report the T-values corresponding to the dummy/parameters between double parentheses. The new values estimated for the mid-point descriptors are all below 0.5 with varying significance. Surprisingly the new mid-point value for the anxiety/depression-dimension is below zero. This may be interpreted as an effect of misspecification due to the linearity assumption.

Table 13.1 Linear model, unrestricted, $x_{2i} = 0.5$, original values

	Average		Median		Mode	
α_0	2.89		-0.09		-5.42	
α_1	20.74	(4.83)	20.88	(4.51)	19.63	(8.08)
α_2	11.70	(4.88)	13.79	(4.55)	9.63	(6.14)
α_3	14.12	(5.78)	14.80	(5.39)	22.43	(7.26)
α_4	14.42	(4.67)	16.12	(4.54)	25.05	(6.13)
α_5	13.77	(4.62)	14.60	(4.30)	13.08	(5.80)
R^2	0.95		0.96		0.94	
degree of freedom	19		19		19	

Table 13.2 Linear model, unrestricted. $x_{2i} = \beta_i$, original values

	Average		Median		Mode	
α_0	12.04		8.83		4.70	
α_1	24.42	(3.38)	23.52	(3.40)	22.12	(4.83)
α_2	15.45	(3.32)	17.46	(3.34)	14.14	(4.74)
α_3	8.45	(3.93)	10.79	(3.95)	18.01	(1.60)
α_4	15.44	(3.35)	17.98	(3.36)	27.84	(4.77)
α_5	8.43	(3.39)	8.84	(3.41)	5.9	(4.84)
β_1	0.13	((-4.28))	0.20	((-3.35))	0.17	((-2.43))
β_2	0.18	((-2.13))	0.15	((-2.66))	0.06	((-1.90))
β_3	0.28	((-1.09))	0.26	((-1.36))	0.20	((-1.99))
β_4	0.19	((-2.08))	0.28	((-1.71))	0.44	((-0.52))
β_5	-0.13	((-3.10))	-0.23	((-2.94))	-0.97	((-2.78))
R2	0.98		0.98		0.98	
degrees of freedom	14		14		14	

In our first estimates, we did not impose any restrictions on our parameters. Now we will assume that α_0, = 0 and $\sum \alpha_i$ = 1. The most important implications of these assumptions are that the value assigned to [11111] is always 100 and that the value assigned to [33333] is always 0. Consequently, we rescaled the observed valuations in a linear way, forcing the upper value at 100 and the lower value at 0. Results are presented in the Tables 13.3 and 13.4.

Again we observe negative estimates for the value of the mid-point descriptor on the anxiety/depression dimension, and considerable differences for the weights assigned to the various dimensions.

As an alternative to taking the central tendency measures, we may use the individual observations as the starting point for our estimations. Minimizing least squares without restrictions on the parameters would result in parameter estimates that are almost identical to the results on the basis of the average values. Differences would be the result of differences in the number of observations to calculate the averages.

Table 13.3 Linear model, restricted, x_{2i} = 0.5, rescaled values

	Average		Median		Mode	
α_0	0		0		0	
α_1	26.24	(10.44)	24.82	(10.24)	21.37	(9.98)
α_2	5.01	(10.25)	6.06	(10.05)	0.60	(9.80)
α_3	30.96	(12.05)	30.70	(11.82)	35.23	(11.52)
α_4	18.82	(10.71)	14.72	(10.50)	27.31	(10.24)
α_5	18.98		18.71		15.30	
R^2	0.76		0.77		0.79	
degree of freedom	21		21		21	

Table 13.4 Linear model, restricted, x_{2i} = β_i rescaled values

	Average		Median		Mode	
α_0	0		0		0	
α_1	31.84	(6.17)	29.32	(5.96)	25.09	(5.64)
α_2	19.47	(6.17)	20.65	(5.96)	15.56	(5.64)

Table 13.4 Linear model, restricted, $x_{2i} = \beta_i$ rescaled values (Continued)

α_3	16.82	(7.07)	17.12	(6.83)	22.21	(8.46)
α_4	17.74	(6.18)	19.73	(5.98)	28.06	(5.65)
	Average		Median		Mode	
α_5	14.12		13.17		9.10	
β_1	0.21	((-2.66))	0.25	((-216))	0.24	((-2.09))
β_2	0.30	((-1.13))	0.22	((-1.75))	0.18	((-1.63))
β_3	0.22	((-1.41))	0.19	((-1.68))	0.18	((-2.31))
β_4	0.07	((-2.08))	0.15	((-2.00))	0.39	((-0.96))
β_5	-0.20	((-2.76))	0.23	((-2.79))	-0.62	((-3.13))
R^2	0.94		0.95		0.96	
degrees of freedom	16		16		16	

As stated before, this is not necessarily true when we rescale the observations of each individual assigning the value 0 to point [33333] and the value 1 to point [11111]. In Table 13.5 we present the results, first with the mid-point descriptors valued at the value 0.5, second by varying that value. Like us, readers should not pay too much attention to the artefactual increase in degrees in freedom and the decrease in R^2.

Table 13.5 Linear model, restricted, all individual values rescaled

	$x_{2i} = 0{,}5$		$x_{2i} = \beta_i$	
α_0	0		0	
α_1	27.35	(0.96)	32.19	(0.84)
α_2	6.28	(0.94)	20.06	(0.84)
α_3	29.16	(1.12)	15.96	(0.97)
α_4	18.83	(0.99)	17.62	(0.85)
α_5	18.40		14.16	
β_1	0.5		0.23	((-18.70))
β_2	0.5		0.32	((-7.79))
β_3	0.5		0.22	((-9.70))
β_4	0.5		0.08	((-16.03))

Table 13.5 Linear model, restricted, all individual values rescaled

β_5	0.5	-0.21	((-20.07))
R^2	0.63	0.74	
degrees of freedom	5875	5870	

Again we observe a negative estimate for the value of the mid-point descriptor on the anxiety/depression dimension. The differences in weights between both models, using the same data, appear to be considerable too.

13.8 THE MULTIPLICATIVE MODEL

Regarding the estimation of the multiplicative models we followed two strategies. First, we concentrated on first order effects. Based on the average values, we included all interactions effect one by one, estimating $4 + 3 + 2 + 1 = 10$ models with seven parameters. The results are presented in Table 13.6. All interaction parameters appear to be positive, which means that a decrease in one dimension affects the valuation more when the health state on the other dimension is better. It is questionable to what extent this is a real phenomenon. We have seen that mid-point values are estimated at values below 0.5 if they are varied. The significant interaction effects may well be the result of mis-specification introduced by the assumption of a value 0.5 for the mid-points.

Table 13.6 Multiplicative model, one first order effect. $x_{2i} = 0.5$, observed values

interaction	α_0	α_1	α_2	α_3	α_4	α_5	$\alpha_i\alpha_j$	R^2	d.o.f.
1/2	8.62	4.41	-1.66	11.85	18.00	9.47	29.97	0.963	18
		7.03	6.25	4.98	4.33	4.21	10.46		
1/3	5.98	11.41	12.59	2.89	14.83	12.85	19.71	0.955	18
		6.77	4.62	8.13	4.59	4.37	10.60		
1/4	6.62	6.20	13.82	12.15	1.30	16.10	25.43	0.964	18
		6.43	4.19	4.93	6.08	3.98	8.68		
1/5	8.48	4.35	9.16	12.10	17.23	1.78	29.10	0.972	18
		5.38	3.67	4.31	3.67	4.51	7.13		
2/3	4.25	20.31	8.51	9.12	15.38	12.58	8.52	0.948	18
		4.94	6.84	9.44	5.15	5.00	12.61		
2/4	5.12	20.55	5.54	14.63	4.65	13.94	15.38	0.953	18
		4.66	6.12	5.58	7.80	4.45	9.79		
2/5	6.28	19.56	3.72	12.78	14.77	5.89	16.37	0.954	18
		4.67	6.67	5.58	4.66	6.45	9.78		

Table 13.6 Multiplicative model, one first order effect. $x_{2i} = 0.5$, observed values

3/4	4.72	19.54	13.05	6.89	7.35	13.58	15.04	0.951	18
		4.83	4.89	7.87	7.17	4.53	11.36		
3/5	6.00	20.00	10.69	4.97	14.45	6.79	17.78	0.955	18
		4.59	4.65	7.45	4.61	5.83	9.84		
4/5	4.35	22.41	11.62	12.84	6.86	6.77	14.80	0.951	18
		4.90	4.78	5.74	7.41	6.93	11.90		

The second strategy was to estimate the first order interaction model by stepwise linear regression. We did this for the original values and for the rescaled values using the individual data. The results, including the main effects, are presented in Table 13.7.

Surprisingly, we see some negative coefficients, but It should be noted that they have no decreasing effects on the value functions at the points under observation. An increase of 0.5 on each dimension increases the value function in all points.

Table 13.7 Multiplicative model, first order effects, stepwise linear regression including main effects

	original values		rescaled values	
α_0	11.91		7.62	
α_1	-3.71	(1.44)	-3.96	(1.47)
α_2	2.34	(1.23)	2.21	(1.28)
α_3	4.58	(1.40)	6.26	(1.52)
α_4	11.33	(1.54)	14.42	(1.86)
α_5	-2.39	(1.25)	2.81	(1.26)
α_{12}	25.08	(2.17)	31.31	(3.03)
α_{13}			-6.39	(3.14)
α_{15}	20.33	(1.64)	23.53	(1.78)
α_{24}	-4.53	(2.06)	-7.58	((2.55)
α_{34}	12.91	(2.08)	17.15	(3.03)
α_{45}	10.03	(2.05)	9.03	(2.24)
R^2	0.77		0.80	
degrees of freedom	5868		5867	

After rescaling the dimensions in a linear way from a [0,1] scale to a [1,3] scale main effects may be left out from the stepwise regression. The value 0 is excluded and the effects of a variable may be expressed through the direct effects themselves as well as through interaction terms. The results are presented in Table 13.8. Again, we note that the negative coefficients do not imply that the value functions decreases while the scores on the dimensions increase. Now, the direct effects of the third and fourth dimension are excluded from the model. Only mobility, self-care and anxiety/depression appear to affect the value function in a direct way. So, pain/discomfort and usual activities only enter the model indirectly.

Table 13.8 Multiplicative model, first order effects, stepwise linear regression

	original values		rescaled values	
α_0	21.21		17.32	
α_1	-12.18	(1.04)	-12.74	(1.06)
α_2	-5.01	(0.95)	5.16	(0.95)
α_5	-7.98	(0.93)	-8.90	(0.93)
α_{12}	5.70	(0.48)	6.19	(0.48)
α_{15}	5.14	(0.38)	5.49	(0.38)
α_{34}	2.82	(0.21)	2,93	(0.21)
α_{45}			248	(0.29)
R^2	0.77		0.80	
degrees of freedom	5871	5867		

The last estimates that we will present here concern the multiplicative model as proposed by Torrance *et al*, 1982. We estimated the model on the basis of the average values rescaled on a [0,1] scale. The parameter estimates are:

$\alpha = 3.7900 \quad (0.01)$

$\alpha_1 = 0.1349 \quad (0.031)$

$\alpha_2 = 0.0840 \quad (0.023)$

$\alpha_3 = 0.0598 \quad (0.026)$

$\alpha_4 = 0.0909 \quad (0.025)$

$\alpha_5 = 0.0897 \quad (0.064)$

As the $\sum \alpha_i$ are less then one and as $\alpha > 0$, all dimensions should be interpreted as complements. This means that an improvement on any one of the dimensions is less useful than a simultaneous improvement on several.

13.9 DISCUSSION

We have used the data from the Rotterdam survey of the EuroQol Group to explore the possibility of estimating a value function on the basis of which one should be able to attach values to health states for which no values are available. We have distinguished between three subjects that are directly related to our main quesion: the choice of a criterium function, the scales of the values and the dimensions and last but not least the specification of the model. We have seen that all three subjects are interrelated by using simple regression techniques.

Using linear models we included parameters allowing us to estimate the values of the mid-point descriptors on our dimension-scales. We observed negative coefficients and draw the conclusion that this was due to mis-specification. Using parameters to model interaction effects, we conclude that the significance of the observed interactions might be due to mis-specifications of the value of the mid-point descriptors. Estimating both effects at the same time would mean that we would have to include at least 5 parameters more, while we would still only have values for 25 health states. This might not be a problem when we use individual data but it will be if we use medians and modes. Also for this purpose it may be fruitful to think about other criterium functions in which more information is used, for example all distances between the various health states. A first step that we will take is to calculate all predictions from all models. The differences might be less than expected on the basis of the differences in parameters. All further additional work is open for discussion. When it comes to making choices taking account of the opinions in all participating centres, we will use a multiplicative model with only one main effect: the Rotterdam variable.

Presented at the EuroQol Plenary Meeting: Lund, Sweden, 1991

13.10 REFERENCE

Torrance G W, Boyle M H, Horwood S P. Application of multi-attribute utility theory to measure social preferences for health states. Opns.Res. 1982;30:1043-1069.

14
Some considerations concerning negative values for EQ-5D health states

Frank de Charro, Jan Busschbach,
Marie-Louise Essink-Bot, Ben van Hout and Paul Krabbe

In this discussion paper we bring together a number of considerations which might be relevant to gain insight into the use of negative values for EQ-5D health states. This seems relevant since the introduction of negative values will inevitably lead to a discussion about these values, and the background to these figures has to be explained and documented. In theory and in practice it is possible to avoid the use of negative values even in cases where states are considered to be worse than death (WTD). However if one prefers to avoid explicit negative values for EQ-5D health states, other issues arise and it seems to us to be important to have an understanding of these issues. It is possible to understand the nature of the issues involved because the results and data of the MVH project are available. We consider this project as a milestone in the work on quality of life measurement and wish to make explicit our admiration for this scientific endeavour. It is only because of this project that the EuroQol Group is in a position to discuss tariffs based on a large empirical study in which several measurement methods were applied. Our discussion is thus to be seen as an effort to gain insight into the subtleties of the subject and we hope to contribute to the fruitful and widespread use of the results of the project.

The issues raised by the negative values for EQ-5D health states are complex and relevant arguments derive from the fields of psychology, statistics, economics, ethics, and political science. Since it is nearly impossible for somebody who is trained in one of these disciplines to have a clear understanding of all the issues, a discussion at the level of the Group seems to be a fruitful way to obtain a fuller picture.

In this paper, the UK Al and A2 tariffs are chosen as a starting point. The results are derived using the Time Trade Off (TTO) method and will be seen by the EuroQol Group and others as nicely fitting into the framework of economic project appraisal. Some elements might also be relevant for VAS tariffs, but for the purposes of this discussion it was decided to concentrate on the Al and A2 tariffs.

14.1 NEGATIVE VALUES

Figure 14.1 shows the untransformed mean and median values for 43 health states, (11111) and 42 states for which data were gathered by means of the TTO method. The values were derived from the transformed individual values by applying $v = v' / (1 + v')$ if $v' < 0$. The states are given numbers from 1 to 43 and sorted on the means of the TTO - outcomes. Only 14 out of 43 health states have a positive mean and so

P. Kind et al. (eds.), EQ-5D concepts and methods, 171–179.

there are 29 negative means. If the median is used there are 12 negative values and thus 31 positive ones. The minimum mean value of the untransformed means is the value -8.9 for state (33333). The corresponding median value is -1,7. The mean and median are both lower then -1.

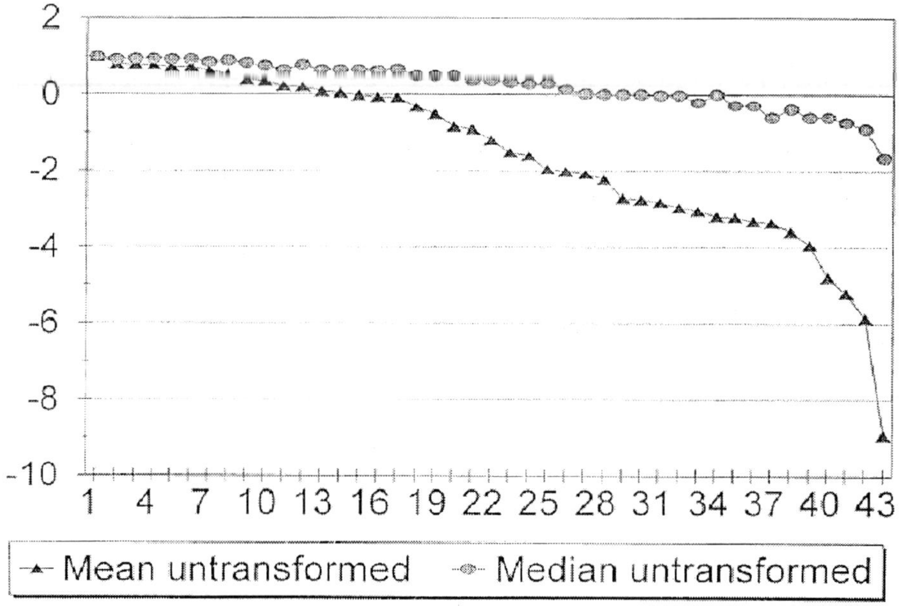

Figure 14.1 Median and mean TTO data

The distribution of the individual values for state (33333) is shown in Figure 14.2, which shows a scatter of the relative frequencies against the non-transformed TTO values. For 19% of the respondents the theoretical extreme values were registered. So 503 out of 2997 respondents scored the theoretical maximum of -39 (which is 9.75/ 0.25). There were 424 respondents (14%) who valued state (33333) in the range from 0 through 1. Among them were 19 respondents who put the value of state (33333) at 1.

In the calculation of the mean these 19 respondents could be counterbalanced by 1 respondent, who would desperately provide a -19. Among the respondents there were 23 of these desperados. Table 14.1 contains the stem leaf plot of the observations for state (33333).

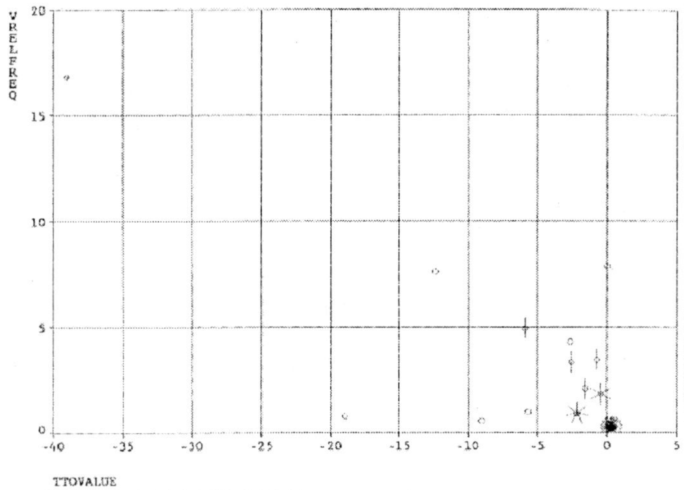

Figure 14.2 TTO 33333 scattered

Table 14.1 Stem leaf plot of the observations for state 33333 (TTO 33333 Stem Leaved)

Valid cases: 2997,0				Missing cases: ,0			Percent missing: ,0
Mean	-8,9102	Std Err	,2556	Min	-39,0000	Skewness	-1 ,5489
Median	-1,6667	Variance	195,8506	Max	1,0000	S E Skew	,0447
5% Trim	-7,7629	Std Dev	13,9947	Range	40,0000	Kurtosis	,6687
				IQR	11,9540	S E Kurt	,0894

Frequency	Stem & Leaf	
503,00	Extremes (-39,0)	
,00	-19	
,00	-18	
23,00	-17	000
,00	-16	
,00	-15	
,00	-14	
,00	-13	
228,00	-12	3333333333333333333333333
,00	-11	
,00	-10	
17,00	-9	00
,00	-8	
137,00	-7	000000000000000
,00	-6	
30,00	-5	666
189,00	-4	000777777777777777777
112,00	-3	000444444444
225,00	-2	0000003336666666666666666
353,00	-1	000000011111112233335566666666666666888
756,00	-0	0000000000111122222222222223333333333444444444444555666666666666666666777778889999999999
405,00	0	000000000000000000000000000000011223344556789
19,00	1	00

Stem width: 1,000

Each leaf: 9 case(s)

14.2 STIMULUS AND RESPONSE

Respondents were given the choice at the beginning of a valuation exercise to choose immediate death instead of being in a state for 10 years and then die. If a respondent then chose immediate death the state to be valued was considered to be WTD. It is difficult to reconstruct what happens exactly in the mind of respondents when confronted with these stimuli. The fear of death is a very powerful psychological motive and this drive might lead to less rational responses. Is it difficult to believe that respondents develop a (rationally perverse) preference for WTD calculation procedures over Better then Death (BTD) procedures? Respondents might be aware after some exercises that it is actually possible to compensate WTD states by full health states and develop a preference for the WTD model. This makes sense if a respondent wants to avoid the confrontation with death. In WTD procedures it is possible to postpone death by compensating with high numbers of full health years. In BTD procedures, death comes nearer and nearer for worse health states.

After this decision the respondent was confronted with a set of special questions intended to generate a TTO value for this health state. In the case of BTD states the health state to be valued was fixed at 10 years to be substituted by an unknown number of years in full health. In the case of WTD states the respondent was led through an exercise which brought him/her to the point of indifference between the time, t, in the WTD state and the compensating time interval, x, in full health. This procedure offered the possibility to use full health as common denominator in valuing both BTD states and WTD states.

The procedure followed provides a negative extreme value since the WTD procedure stops if the respondent has chosen a value of -39. This is the consequence of undertaking the TTO exercise in quarter-year steps. So the minimum time for t would be 0.25 year and for x 0.9.75 and minus the ratio between x and t would be -39. The time interval used is arbitrary and smaller time intervals generate higher maximum extreme values. In the calculation of the mean the influence of these extreme responses might rise accordingly. So the means of the values of WTD states are sensitive for the arbitrarily chosen time intervals and cannot be considered as objective values. The theoretical minimum time interval would be zero seconds to be compensated by 10 years minus 0 seconds. The resulting minimum TTO value would be minus infinite. It is impossible to use this value in health state appraisals where state (33333) years have to be compensated by years in better health states with a maximum value of +1, unless there was an infinite number of those years.

To be able to standardize on full health years a compensating time framework was used. The respondents were asked to distribute a time span of 10 years over a period t in the WTD state and a compensating time x = (10 - t) in full health. This procedure is different from the BTD procedure where the state to be valued is constantly perceived as lasting 10 years. So each value of a WTD state relates to a different time span t. This is unavoidable since fixing time at 10 years in a time framework where compensation by more than

10 years would be possible would lead to very high compensating intervals, such as 40 years. This would often be incompatible with the life expectancy of the respondent. Moreover the resulting trade-offs would become incomparable with the outcomes of the BTD procedures. How certain can we be, however, that this incompatibility does not exist in the constant sum procedure applied in the MVH study?

14.3 EXTREME VALUES MODERATED

The results from the TTO exercise will be very appealing for economists, since the concept links nicely into the framework of health programme evaluation and cost-effectiveness analysis. The negative values generated by the WTD procedures are, however, potentially embarrassing and the high proportion of extremes will create doubts about the acceptability of their use. So before using the negative values for modeling exercises, these values have been transformed using the formula: v' = v / (1 - v), where v is the value resulting from the TTO exercise for a respondent and v' is the transformed value. The resulting transformed values lie on an interval from 0 to -1. Figure 14.3 presents a graph which shows the transformed mean and median for the health states included in the MVH study. The untransformed means and medians are also included in the graph. The transformed means are much higher then the untransformed means and the differences increase for the WTD health states. In fact it seems that the transformed means follow rather closely the pattern of the medians. However, in the severe WTD states the untransformed medians are lower then the transformed means.

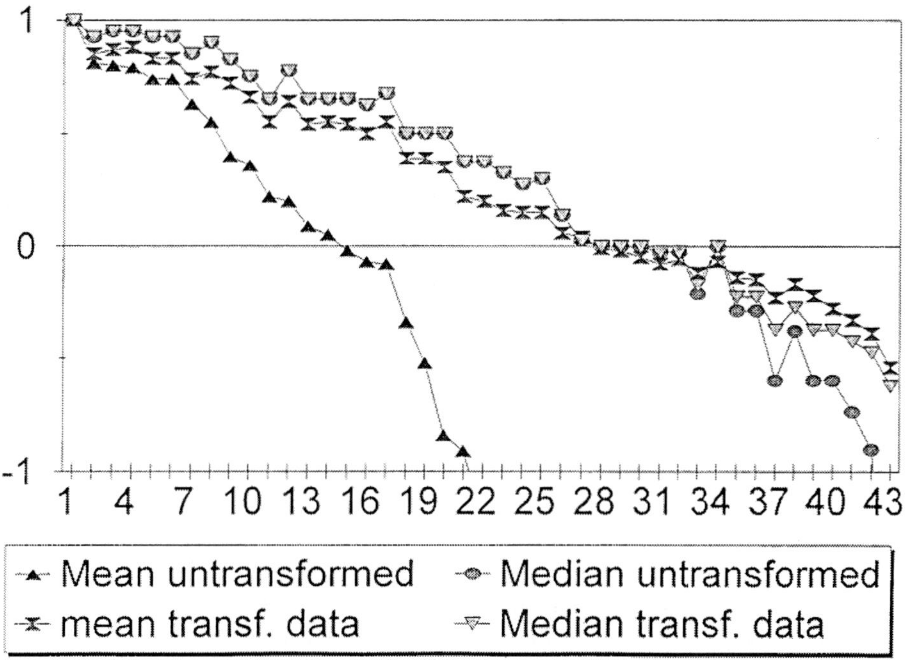

Figure 14.3 Plus transformation

The models are estimated on data which have been transformed in the cases where the TTO valuations were negative. However the values resulting from the transformation are not transformed back afterwards. The combination of the transformed negative values with the positive untransformed values assumes that the transformed negative values reflect utilities in the same way as the positive values. It is to be expected that the scientific debate on this topic might be intense, since at first sight it is not easy to understand that transformed negative outcomes of TTO studies are to be considered as utilities. Patrick wrote in Medical Decision Making about the transformation used in the MVH study and concluded that "the transformed values should not be interpreted as utilities" (Patrick *et al*, 1994). The method used to value the negative WTD states implies that the respondent has to find a point of indifference under the constraint that the sum of t and x is a constant sum, 10. Poulton appears to be critical of this Constant Sum Method and prefers a method of ratio scaling (Poulton, 1989). It seems that there is still no a standard method which can be used to deal with WTD states.

But perhaps the method used does not generate a bias since the units used are familiar to the respondents. In that case a transformation would be superfluous. However if one expects that the Constant Sum Method generates a bias, it is not easy to explain why the transformation used is a necessary and sufficient method to correct for this. It has to be expected that many potential users of the EQ-5D will be afraid to apply a tariff which has serious conceptual flaws.

The transformation results in a maximum negative value of minus 1 for a health state. If one accepts the use of negative values there is no reason why those values have to be bounded by minus 1. Why would a period in a certain health state not be bad enough to be compensated by more than that period in full health?

14.4 MEAN - MEDIAN

Economic theory does not provide a generally applicable rule for the use of either the mean or the median. The mean might be appropriate since it reflects the intensity of the preference of the consumers of a health care programme and the median might be appropriate since it reflects favourite rule of decision-making in democratic environments. Choosing the mean implies that data at the individual level can be used.

There is no special reason why the extreme value for the mean (-8.91) would be unacceptable. However if one judges a transformation to be necessary to moderate the extremes, then the use of the median is a direct way to do this, since the median neglects the intensity of the judgments of respondents.

The application of the mean does give a very strong influence on the resulting values for respondents who are at the extremes. It could be argued that this is not in line with the practice of cost-effectiveness analysis, where the effectiveness of a programme is measured by counting life years under the assumption that all human life years have the same weight. The analogue of this would be that values for the quality of life years are determined using the same rule and this implies the use of the median. Moreover the extreme values are not justified in any way by real behaviour, since the respondents have only to say that they judge a WTD state at the extreme, they do not have to take the consequences.

By the use of the median, important weaknesses that have to be dealt with when using means are avoided. In fact, the distributions hardly justify the use non-normalized data. It is not necessary to transform the data. The median reflects the one (wo)man one vote majority rule, which is widely accepted.

14.5 DISCUSSION

Figure 14.4 contains two variants of median values. In addition to the values for the original medians, the rescaled values of the median on a 0 - 1 scale are shown, where 1 is full health, state (11111), and 0 is the value of state (33333).

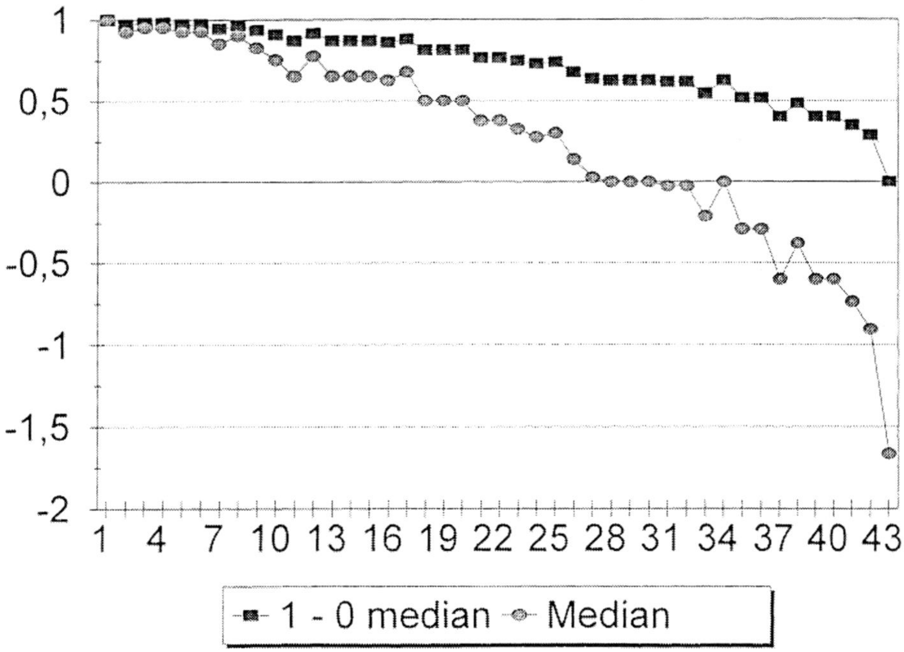

Figure 14.4 Two medians

In both versions of the median values there is a strong reward for health programmes that enable a transition from states such as (33333), (33323), (33232) which are the health states at the lower end of the valuation spectrum. The difference is that in the rescaled version of the median, the explicit use of negative values is avoided.

A disadvantage of rescaling to a scale between zero and 1 is that the value for state (33333) is put at 0 and so programmes which generate only life years in state (33333) generate no QALYs. This is not easy to explain. Moreover the implicit valuation of death would be approximately 0.6 and this is intuitively a very high value. If this implicit value for death is not used in scenario calculations then the ranking of scenarios on QALYs gained may differ between the case where the original medians are used and the case where the rescaled medians are used.

The advantage of using rescaled medians would be that negative values are totally avoided. For some people, clinicians and policymakers, the notion of negative quality of life values is unacceptable and the result might be that indices for quality of life are not used at all. The resistance to these values might be strengthened by methodological questions which have still to be answered, especially with respect to the Constant Sum Method and the transformation.

Negative values imply that life in certain heath states is unliveable. It is well known that the judgment of people who are in these health states differs significantly from the judgment of healthy people. Many times patients in extremely bad health states have a desire for life which is very strong. There is much to be said in favour of the judgments of healthy people for valuations of health states in cases where the patients might be underestimating their need for health care because of coping behaviour. However there might be a need for more discussion about neglecting patients' judgment in cases where healthy people judge a state to be negative in value and the people in that state judge it positively (or positively enough not to commit suicide).

The framework in which decisions are made, based on indices for quality of life, has not been sufficiently discussed. It is considered by many to be outside the realm of science. There is a vague understanding that application at the level of intra-program comparisons is not problematic, since decisions made in this framework concern mostly resource allocation and the different programme alternatives are understood by the decision-makers. There is probably also a common understanding that physicians should be careful in applying indices of quality of life in individual cases. In cases where EQ-5D values become negative, the considerations involved should be made explicit. If we abstain from this others might consider negative QALY values to be a plea for euthanasia. This is not what the EuroQol Group is advocating.

It might be wise to encourage simultaneous use of TTO values with negative values for some ranges of health states and some other set of values with only positive values. The positive set might be the set of rescaled medians, but may also be a set of values derived from the VAS scaling exercise. In cost-effectiveness studies these sets of values do not often produce conflicting values and so simultaneous use increases the acceptability of the research results. Sometimes scenarios require the application of negative values, but in these cases the availability of additional information from other scales obliges researchers to argue their case and maximize the understanding of their research

Presented at the EuroQol Plenary Meeting: Barcelona, Spain, 1995

14.6 REFERENCES

Patrick D, Starks H, Cain K, et al. Measuring preferences for health states worse than death. Medical Decision Making 1994;14(l):9-18.

Poulton E C. Bias in quantifying judgments. Lawrence Erbaum Associates ltd. Publishers, 1989:51.

15
Health states considered worse than 'being dead'

Stefan Björk and Rikard Althin

15.1 BACKGROUND

A number of empirical studies have indicated that there are health states worse than death (Rosser and Kind, 1978; Kind and Rosser, 1979; Sintonen, 1981; Sutherland *et al*, 1982; Torrance *et al*, 1982; Torrance, 1984). As 'being dead', for obvious reasons, is often chosen as the reference point and bottom endpoint (i.e. the state to which the lowest value on the scale is attached) on a health-status measurement scale, a health index or a quality of life scale, these results have highlighted some central questions.

One basic assumption in multiattribute utility analysis (MAUT) (Keeney and Raifa, 1976) is utility independence between health status and life years (Keeney, 1974). This assumption will be strongly questionned if the empirical results are valid (Pliskin *et al*, 1980). It then seems that one, *prima facie*, has to reject either this basic assumption in MAUT or the results of a number of empirical studies. Torrance and Feeny (1989) propose that health states considered worse than death be equal to death, i.e. to have the weight 0.

In this paper we present yet another study where some health states are considered to be worse than 'being dead' (Brooks *et al*, 1991). The study is a part of the development work of the EuroQol Group (Euroqol Group, 1990). The objectives of this paper are twofold: to scrutinize how valid the evaluation of the state 'being dead' is according to a Swedish study and to present a proposed solution for dealing with health states considered worse than 'being dead'.

15.2 METHOD

We used a sample of 1000 Swedish individuals (Brooks *et al*, 1991). 349 of those responded to a health-status measurement questionnaire developed by the EuroQol Group (Euroqol Group, 1990). The 349-group was divided into two subgroups; the 141-group including those who did not answer all questions and the 208-group including those who answered all questions. We compared the mean value of the two groups' evaluations of thirteen health states and of 'being dead'. A description of the health states was presented in a two-sheet questionnaire where the respondents were asked to rate eight states on each sheet. The first sheet is presented in figure 15.1. Four variables - age, sex, education and worked in health/social service - were used to test if the evaluation of 'being dead' and of the health states differed by variable.

P. Kind et al. (eds.), EQ-5D concepts and methods, 181–189.

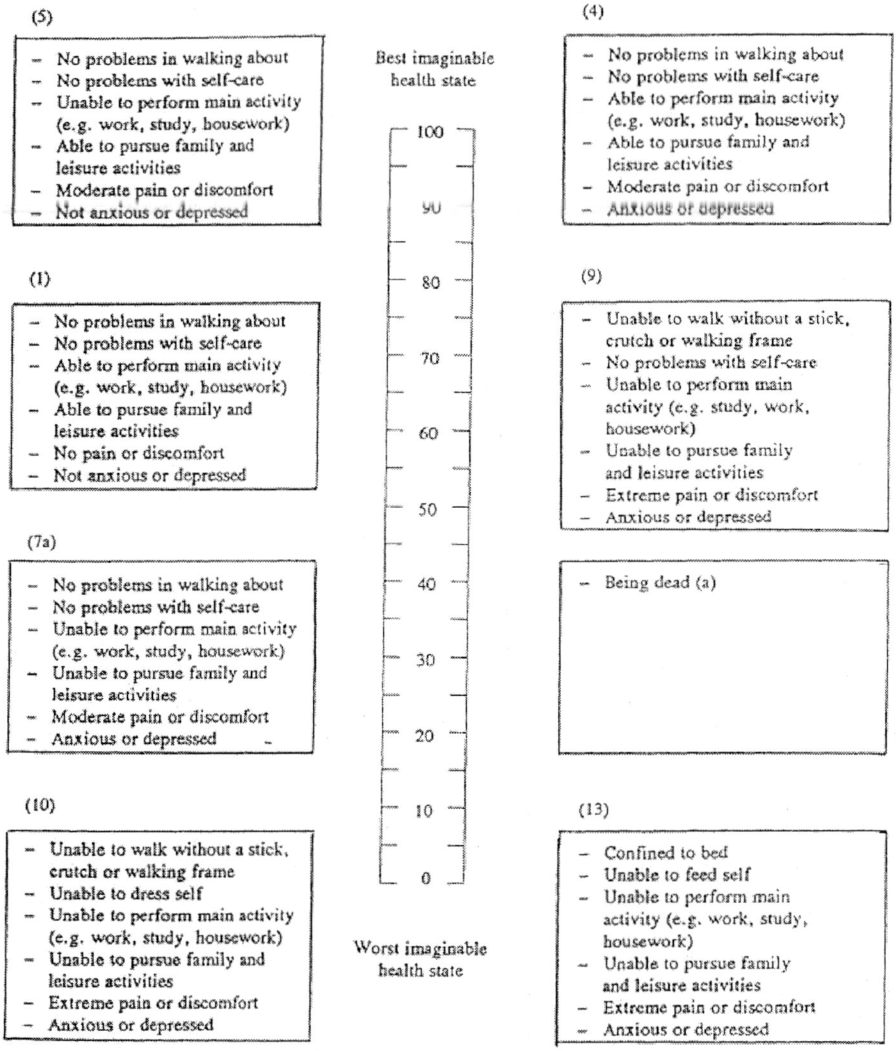

(5)
- No problems in walking about
- No problems with self-care
- Unable to perform main activity (e.g. work, study, housework)
- Able to pursue family and leisure activities
- Moderate pain or discomfort
- Not anxious or depressed

(1)
- No problems in walking about
- No problems with self-care
- Able to perform main activity (e.g. work, study, housework)
- Able to pursue family and leisure activities
- No pain or discomfort
- Not anxious or depressed

(7a)
- No problems in walking about
- No problems with self-care
- Unable to perform main activity (e.g. work, study, housework)
- Unable to pursue family and leisure activities
- Moderate pain or discomfort
- Anxious or depressed

(10)
- Unable to walk without a stick, crutch or walking frame
- Unable to dress self
- Unable to perform main activity (e.g. work, study, housework)
- Unable to pursue family and leisure activities
- Extreme pain or discomfort
- Anxious or depressed

Best imaginable health state

100 90 80 70 60 50 40 30 20 10 0

Worst imaginable health state

(4)
- No problems in walking about
- No problems with self-care
- Able to perform main activity (e.g. work, study, housework)
- Able to pursue family and leisure activities
- Moderate pain or discomfort
- Anxious or depressed

(9)
- Unable to walk without a stick, crutch or walking frame
- No problems with self-care
- Unable to perform main activity (e.g. study, work, housework)
- Unable to pursue family and leisure activities
- Extreme pain or discomfort
- Anxious or depressed

- Being dead (a)

(13)
- Confined to bed
- Unable to feed self
- Unable to perform main activity (e.g. work, study, housework)
- Unable to pursue family and leisure activities
- Extreme pain or discomfort
- Anxious or depressed

Figure 15.1 The first sheet of the EuroQol valuation exercise

Age was divided into five categories: (1) 15-30 years, (2) 31-45 years, (3) 46-60 years, (4) 61-75 years, (5) 76- and upwards. Education was divided into three categories: (1) minimum schooling, (2) intermediate, (3) higher/degree level. Worked in health/social service was divided into two categories; (1) yes, (2) no. 'Being dead' and one health state occur twice marked (a) and (b) as a test of consistency. This test is not analysed or commented upon in this paper.

To test if the 141-group evaluated 'being dead' and the health states differently from the 208-group, we used a t-test. To test if the evaluation of 'being dead' and if the health states differed within a variable, we used analysis of variance.

Table 15.1 Mean, standard deviation and P-value for evaluation of the health states and 'being dead' by the 141-group and the 208-group

	141-Group		208-Group		
Health State	Mean	Stdev	Mean	Stdev	P-value
1	89.24 (66)	17.05	93.33 (208)	12.74	0.076
2	82.92 (67)	18.00	83.26 (208)	15.52	0.890
3	66.45 (65)	25.28	69.20 (208)	20.99	0.427
4	61.33 (66)	21.67	60.93 (208)	21.59	0.895
5	66.75 (68)	18.99	64.41 (208)	20.03	0.386
6	55.17 (65)	22.59	50.75 (208)	21.02	0.165
7 (a)	36.75 (67)	22.96	35.80 (208)	19.62	0.763
7 (b)	40.29 (62)	23.41	38.05 (208)	19. 30	0.493
8	36.12 (65)	26.33	36.07 (208)	19.89	0.989
9	31.43 (68)	24.86	25.88 (208)	20.11	0.098
10	16.17 (66)	20.46	14.23 (208)	19.22	0.530
11	14.52 (64)	24.03	12.13 (208)	19.36	0.470
Dead (a)	9.77 (30)	19.16	10.45 (208)	24.26	0.861
Dead (b)	9.55 (29)	18.59	10.02 (208)	23.45	0.903
12	12.32 (63)	24.71	8.91 (208)	17.54	0.311
13	11.66 (67)	23.84	7.88 (208)	18.61	0.238

Note: Given in brackets are the number of respondents evaluating a particular health state

15.3 RESULTS

We did not find any statistically significant differences between the 141-group and the 208-group in the evaluation of 'being dead' and of the health states (Table 15.1 and Figure 15.2). By statistical significance we mean significance at the five-percentage level. This implies that the two groups could be put together when looking for differences in age, sex, education and working in the health/social service. The subsequent analysis was carried out for the 349-group. In the first part of the results we present the evaluation of 'being dead' and in the second part the evaluation of health states.

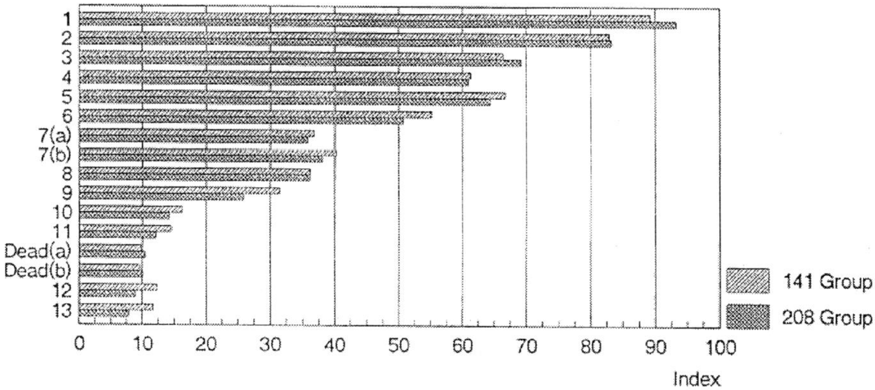

Figure 15.2 The evaluation of health states

Part 1.

Age. There was no statistically significant difference between the five categories of age and the ratings of 'being dead' (Table 15.2). The mean value of 'being dead' ranged from 5.7 (31-45 years) to 14.2 (46-60 years) for (a) and from 5.7 (31-45 years) to 13.8 (61-75 years) for (b).

Table 15.2 P-value for the comparison of 'being dead' and age

	Age					
Health State	16-30	31-45	46-60	61-75	76 >	P-value
Dead (a)	11.12	5.71	14.19	13.64	8.57	0.302
Dead (b)	12.61	5.73	10.23	13.79	8.50	0.361

Sex. In one of the two ratings of 'being dead' (b) there was a statistically significant difference between male and female (Table 15.3). On average, males rated 'being dead' (b) as 13.30 while females rated the same status as 7.22. The other rating of 'being dead' (a) varied from 12.82 (male) to 8.29 (female) and the difference was not statistically significant.

Table 15.3 P-value for the comparison of 'being dead' and sex

	Sex		
Health State	Male	Female	P-value
Dead (a)	12.82	8.29	0.142
Dead (b)	13.30	7.22	0.041

Education. With regard to education, there was no statistically significant difference in the valuation of 'being dead' (Table 15.4). The analysis of variance test was conducted on different levels of education - within each state of 'being dead' ((a) and (b)). 'Being dead' (a) ranged from 8.1 (intermediate) to 13.1 (minimum schooling). 'Being dead' (b) ranged from 9.0 (intermediate) to 12.2 (university).

Table 15.4 P-value for the comparison of 'being dead' and education

	Education			
Health State	Minimum	Intermediate	University	P-value
Dead (a)	12.98	8.14	12.29	0.349
Dead (b)	9.29	9.01	12.20	0.638

Worked in health/social service. There was no statistically significant difference in the evaluation of 'being dead' between those who worked in health/social service and those who did not (Table 15.5). Those not working in the health/social service rated 'being dead' (a) and (b) lower.

Table 15.5 P-value for the comparison of 'being dead' and worked in health/social service

	Worked in health/social service		
Health State	Yes	No	P-value
Dead (a)	10.93	10.17	0.816
Dead (b)	9.44	9.40	0.988

Part 2.

Age. There was a statistically significant difference for seven of the fourteen health states (Table 15.6).

Sex. In four out of fourteen of the health states there was a statistically significant difference (Table 15.6).

Education. In ten out of fourteen health states, there was a statistically significant difference in the evaluation of the health states (Table 15.6).

Working in the health/social service. No statistically significant differences were found regarding work in the health/social service (Table 15.6).

Table 15.6 P-value for the comparison of the evaluation of the health states and 'being dead'

Health State	Age	Sex	Education	Worked in Health/ Social Services
1	0.000	0.001	0.000	0.185
	(274)	(274)	(273)	(271)
2	0.153	0.658	0.663	0.402
	(275)	(275)	(274)	(272)
3	0.823	0.618	0.891	0.532
	(273)	(273)	(272)	(270)
4	0.330	0.663	0.155	0.078
	(274)	(274)	(273)	(271)
5	0.178	0.647	0.021	0.460
	(276)	(276)	(275)	(273)
6	0.283	0.605	0.040	0.866
	(273)	(273)	(272)	(270)
7(a)	0.004	0.715	0.035	0.757
	(275)	(275)	(274)	(272)
7(b)	0.018	0.963	0.048	0.324
	(270)	(270)	(269)	(267)
8	0.002	0.739	0.003	0.886
	(273)	(273)	(272)	(270)
9	0.013	0.934	0.000	0.583
	(276)	(276)	(275)	(273)
10	0.013	0.027	0.051	0.791
	(274)	(274)	(273)	(271)
11	0.151	0.031	0.042	0.545
	(272)	(272)	(271)	(269)
Dead (a)	0.302	0.142	0.349	0.816
	(238)	(238)	(236)	(235)
Dead (b)	0.361	0.041	0.638	0.400
	(237)	(237)	(236)	(234)
12	0.175	0.139	0.015	0.988
	(271)	(271)	(270)	(268)
13	0.035	0.060	0.002	0.626
	(275)	(275)	(274)	(271)

Note: Given in brackets are the numbers of respondents

15.4 DISCUSSION

There was no difference between the 141-group and the 208-group in the evaluation of the health states. Respondents who omitted the evaluation of a particular health state or of 'being dead' (i.e. the 141-group), did not evaluate other health states differently from those who answered all items. Hence, whatever the reason may be for omitting some items of the questionnaire, it did not, according to our study, affect the evaluation of the other health states.

The results of our study do not confirm any difference in the evaluation of 'being dead' according to the variables age, education and working in the health/social sevice. For sex there was, however, a statistically significant difference for 'being dead' (b). On the other hand, our results imply that there were differences in the evaluation of health states according to age, sex and, in particular, to education. The evaluation of 'being dead' was, then, more uniform than the evaluation of different health states. This indicates that the evaluation of 'being dead' was at least as sound as the evaluation of health states.

Presupposing that a uniform evaluation among respondents is to be preferred, and that a low response rate (c.f. the 141-group in Table 15.1) is less important, 'being dead' is, *prima facie*, more suitable to serve as a reference point than health states rated lower than 'being dead'. On the other hand according to empirical results people actually do evaluate some health states as ' worse' than 'being dead'. This means that the reference point 'being dead', according to empirical results, is not synonymous with the bottom endpoint of the scale.

These results mean great problems in measuring changes in health status over time. Health status and life years spent in a health state considered worse than 'being dead', apparently, are considered together, in conflict with the presupposition of utility independence, and a decision is made whether to live or to die (to put it drastically). The basic problem is that 'being dead' is irreversible. A dead person cannot choose (!) to change his/her health (or lack of health) state. So, with the objective of increasing health, 'being dead' is a problem when rated higher than some health states. Even if it were (medically) possible to increase a health state worse than 'being dead', the preference of 'being dead' rules out the actual choice to increase that health state, provided that one has to follow strictly the implications of the evaluation.

Our proposed solution to part of the problem is to apply the well-known distinction between acute and chronic health states. There are two crucial decisions to be made.
1) Fix a probability of an increase of the health state rated lower than 'being dead'.
2) Fix a time limit, for how long a time is it 'better' to endure being in that health state than to rigidly follow the literal recommendation derived from the evaluation of the health states and die. The answers to these two questions will serve as a 'rule of

thumb' distinction for chronic and acute health states, even though there may be very long-lasting acute health states considered worse than 'being dead'.

The more chronic the health state rated lower than 'being dead' is, the more valid the recommendation (to not endure staying alive) is, derived from the empirical results, And vice versa: the more acute the health state the less valid is the recommendation. This is also supported by the findings by Sutherland and colleagues that the increase of the duration of a 'bad' health state also increased the probability to evaluate that state as ' worse' than 'being dead' (Sutherland *et al*, 1982).

It seems that in addition to the distinction between acute and chronic health states, the probability of becoming better then 'being dead' has to be considered when deciding whether or not to follow the recommendation of the empirical results. When there is a sufficiently high probability of recovering and improving that health state, it seems reasonable to make an exception from the empirical results that there are health states worse than 'being dead'. The proposed solution in this paper has, in our opinion, the advantage compared to Torrance and Feeny's proposal that it takes the empirical results seriously.

To sum up, we have suggested a way of combining empirical results with theoretical presuppositions or axioms. Two inferences are, in our opinion, rather well-motivated.

Enduring health states 'worse than death' when they are acute is not inconsistent with having 'being dead' as a reference point which is not synonymous with the bottom endpoint. Provided that the temporary loss of quality of life is less than the future gain in quality of life in staying alive. This means that the reference point may have a 'higher' value on the scale than the bottom endpoint. We suggest that the reference point does not necessarily have to be equal to the bottom endpoint. We then can accept even worse health states than what we know today without having to revise our scale.

If the health state 'worse than death' is chronic the empirical studies provide strong arguments against the assumption of utility independence between life years and health states.

Presented at the EuroQol Plenary Meeting: Lund, Sweden, 1991

15.5 REFERENCES

Brooks R G, Jendteg S, Lindgren B, Persson U, Björk S. Euroqol: Health-related quality of life measurement. Results of the Swedish questionnaire exercise. Health Policy. 1991;18(1):37-48.

Euroqol Group. Euroqol: A new facility for the measurement of health-related quality of life. Health Policy. 1990;16:199-208.
Keeney R L. Multiplicative utility functions. Opns. Res. 1974;22:22-34.

Keeney R L, Raifa H. Decisions with multiple objectives: Preferences and value tradeoffs. New York: John Wiley and Sons, 1976.

Kind P, Rosser R. Death and dying: scaling of death for health status indices. In: Lindberg D A B, Reichertz P L, editors. Lecture notes in medical information. Berlin: Springer-Verlag, 1979:28-36.

Pliskin J, Shepard D, Weinstein H. Utility functions for life years and health status. Opns.Res. 1980:206-224.

Rosser R, Kind P. A scale of valuations of states of illness: Is there a social consensus? International Journal of Epidemiology 1978;7:347-358.

Sintonen H. An approach to measuring and valuing health states. Soc Sci Med 1981;15C:55-65.

Sutherland H J, Llewellyn-Thomas H, Boyd N F, Till J E. Attitudes toward quality of survival: the concept of 'maximum endurable time'. Medical Decision Making 1982;2:299-309.

Torrance G W, Boyle M H, Horwood S P. Application of multi-attribute utility theory to measure social preferences for health states. Opns. Res. 1982;30:1043-1069.

Torrance G W. Health states worse than death. In: Eimeren W van, Engelbrecht R, Flagle C D, editors. 3rd International conference on system science in health care. Berlin: Springer-Verlag, 1984:1085-1089.

Torrance G W, Feeny D. Utilities and quality-adjusted life years. Int J of Technology Assessment in Health Care. 1989;5:559-575.

16
The effect of duration on the values given to the EuroQol states

Arto Ohinmaa and Harri Sintonen

16.1 INTRODUCTION

The EuroQol measure was developed through the cooperation of several European research groups (EuroQol Group, 1990). The measure consists of five dimensions which are: mobility, self-care, usual activities, pain or discomfort and anxiety or depression. Every dimension is divided into three levels:

(i) no problems in the dimension (level 1),
(ii) some or moderate problems in the dimension (level 2), and
(iii) unable to do something or having extreme problems in the dimension (level 3) (Rosser and Sintonen, 1993).

The EuroQol measure will be valued in each country by a population sample. The EuroQol Group has decided to use the Category Rating (CR) method in the valuations. The advantage of the CR method is that it is possible to use it in postal surveys, which makes it an inexpensive and quick way of obtaining national EuroQol index values. However, there are some methodological questions that need further research. One of these is the influence of duration of the states on the values given these states. In the Finnish EuroQol survey three different durations were used: one year, ten years, and an unspecified duration (see Appendix 16.1, page 4). In addition, in a convenience sample the same respondents considered for three different durations: one year, ten years, and one month. In this paper valuations of states with different durations and different methods of valuing the health states are compared.

16.2 DATA AND METHODS

The Finnish EuroQol valuation questionnaires (N = 4000) were sent in November 1992 to randomly selected persons in Finland. The sample was divided into 17 sub-samples and each sub-sample (N = 230) received a different valuation form for completion. Three sub-samples received the standard EuroQol questionnaire (Appendix 16.1, pages 5 and 6), which differed between the groups only in the duration of the states defined on page 4 (Appendix 16.1).

The response rates and the rates of usable responses in the groups are presented in Table 16.1. The response rate was highest in the 'one year' sample (70%) and lowest in the 'ten years' sample (60%). A considerable proportion of the responses were not

P. Kind et al. (eds.), EQ-5D concepts and methods, 191–199.

usable in the analysis. Reasons for this were: 1) the valuation form was returned completely unfilled, 2) only a few health states were valued, and 3) the valuation form included several inconsistent valuations. In particular the values for the logically 'best state' (state 11111) and for the 'worst state' (state 33333) were required to be ranked in that way. The only exceptions were the state 'unconscious' and the state 'death' . In the 'one year' sample 69% of responses were completed appropriately (48% of the whole sample). In this respect the 'ten years' sample gave the worst responses because 59% of the responses were usable (36% of the sample) (Table 16.1). However, these differences were not statistically significant.

Table 16.1 Response rates, and the rate of usable responses in the sub-samples (N = 230 each)

Duration (sub-sample)	Responses		Usable responses		Usable responses of the sample	
	N	%	N	%	N	%
1 year	160	70%	111	69%	111	48%
10 years	139	60%	82	59%	82	36%
Unspecified	152	66%	96	63%	96	42%

Around 50% of the respondents were male. There were no significant differences in rejected responses between the genders. Table 16.2 shows the distribution of respondents by age groups in each sub-sample before and after rejecting the inconsistent responses, and the percentage of the responses that were rejected in each age group. It can be seen that nearly 50% of the final data came from the youngest age group (18-35 years). The percentage of rejected responses grew significantly (P = 0.000) in every sub-sample with increasing age.

Table 16.2 The distribution of respondents by age groups in each sub-sample before and after rejection of inconsistent responses and the percentage of the rejected responses

	1 year			10 years			Unspecified		
Age	Responses Rejected			Responses Rejected			Responses Rejected		
group	N	%	Usable	N	%	Usable	N	%	Usable
18-35	57	9%	52	45	11%	40	48	4%	46
36-50	32	10%	29	23	35%	15	22	27%	16
51-65	18	22%	14	27	74%	7	23	52%	11
65-80	53	70%	16	43	53%	20	59	61%	23
Total	160		111	138		82	152		96

The second set of data came from a convenience sample where the respondents filled out the standard EuroQol valuation form. In the questionnaire the first six pages were from the original valuation form. On pages seven and eight the page six health states were replicated and the introductory text on the upper part of the page was the following: "On this page the same health states are presented as on the previous page. You should now think that every health state lasts for 10 years (one month). What happens after that is not known and should not be taken into account." Before the valuation, the task was briefly introduced to the respondents and in addition the different durations were mentioned. It was stated that if the duration was not important they could use the same values on pages 6, 7 and 8. If the duration changed their values for health states, they could do this in any way they liked. They were also free to change the value of the state 'dead' for each duration.

The convenience sample consisted of 60 respondents who had been to an introductory course of lectures in health economics in Northern Finland. 75% of the respondents worked in the health care sector and 80% of them were female. The mean age in the sample was 39 years. Although the sample is not from the 'general population', it can still give some information about the influence of duration on health state values. In particular, it gives the possibility to study the question: do respondents change their values when the same health states are presented with different durations?

16.3 RESULTS

The mean and median values for the states in the Finnish EuroQol survey are shown in Table 16.3. The different health states are presented in the form of 5 digit codes, in which the first number refers to the dimension 'mobility', the second to 'self-care', the third to 'usual activities', the fourth to 'pain or discomfort' and the fifth to 'anxiety or depression'. Level 1 means that there are no problems in the dimension, level 2 means that there are some problems and level 3 means that there are severe problems in the dimension

Table 16.3 The mean and median values of different health states in the Finnish EuroQol survey when their duration is defined to be 1 year, 10 years or unspecified

Health	1 year		10 years		Unspecified	
state	mean	median	mean	median	mean	median
11111a)	95.7	99.0	96.6	100.0	95.1	99.0
11111b)	96.2	99.0	96.5	100.0	95.1	99.5
21111	77.3	80.0	78.4	80.0	77.8	80.0
12111	64.8	70.0	67.4	71.5	65.5	70.0
11211	77.8	80.0	81.0	82.0	79.9	80.0
11121	73.6	79.0	77.8	80.0	77.5	80.0
11112	60.4	62.0	62.6	64.5	67.6	70.0
11122	46.2	50.0	47.3	50.0	50.7	50.0
32211	39.7	40.0	40.4	41.0	40.9	40.0
21232	35.6	39.0	37.1	39.0	40.1	36.5

Table 16.3 The mean and median values of different health states in the Finnish EuroQol survey when their duration is defined to be 1 year, 10 years or unspecified (Continued)

Health	1 year		10 years		Unspecified	
state	mean	median	mean	median	mean	median
33321	18.7	19.0	21.2	20.0	22.0	20.0
22233	27.8	25.0	27.1	23.5	30.3	30.0
22323	23.2	20.0	23.1	20.0	22.2	20.0
33333a)	6.9	3.0	7.3	5.0	8.6	3.0
33333b)	8.0	5.0	8.7	5.0	9.2	4.0
nconsc.	5.5	0.0	4.8	1.5	9.0	2.0
dead a)	10.8	1.0	11.4	0.0	10.3	3.0
dead b)	11.2	0.5	9.0	0.5	11.4	4.0

Table 16.3 shows that there were no big systematic differences in the valuations between the sub-samples with different durations. In addition, measured by 95% confidence intervals, the means in each sub-sample did not differ significantly from each other. When the mean and the median values for the states are compared, it can be seen that these values were usually quite close to each other. The biggest differences between these values were in the state 'death' This result was also expected, because nearly half of the respondents gave a value of zero to the state 'death', while some subjects valued it at even more than 50. The state 'death' was also found to be difficult to value, since about 23% of respondents who gave usable values to the other states had not answered or had inconsistent values for the state 'death'. One cause of rejection was that the state 'death' was valued to be the best health state or it received a value of 100.

The values obtained for the convenience sample are presented in Table 16.4. The differences between the durations were compared by taking 95% confidence intervals from the mean values. It can be seen that respondents changed their values significantly on the health states in seven states of the nine when the durations were ten years and one month. Between one year and ten years only the value of the state 32211 changed, and between one year and one month the state 33333 had different mean values at the 95% confidence interval. The logic for the mean values is the following: except for the states 11111 and 'dead' the ten years values are the lowest, then the one year values are a little higher, and finally the one month values are higher than the previous two. The state 'dead' is valued such that the 'zero point' rises when the duration increases. This means that if the state 'dead' is used as an anchor in scale transformations, the differences between the durations would be even wider.

The difference between the two sets of data is quite clear. When the duration is stated only on the page 4, it seems to affect valuations (Table 16.3). When emphasis is put on the duration, it seems to have systematic effects on the values (Table 16.4).

Table 16.4 Mean values and 95% confidence intervals in the convenience sample where the same respondents valued health states during one year, ten years and one month time periods (N = 60)

Health state	One year	Ten years	One month
11111	95.7	97.1	97.1
	94.3-97.1	96.0-98.9	96.0-98.9
21111*)	82.2	80.5	87.2
	79.4-85.0	77.7-83.3	84.7-89.7
12111	73 . 0	72 . 1	76.0
	68.5-77.5	67.5-76.7	72.1-79.9
11112*)	58.6	50.9	61.9
	54.5-62.7	46.6-55.2	57.4-66.4
32211**)	51.9	42.2	55.9
	47.9-55.9	37.9-46.5	51.1-60.7
22323*)	21.8	18 . 0	25.4
	18.4-25.2	14.6-21.4	21.6-29.2
33333**)	8.3	6.3	17.1
	5.7-10.9	4.0-8.6	13 .0-21.2
Uncon. *)	10 . 7	4.9	16.6
	5.8-15.6	1.4-8.4	11.2-22.0
Dead *)	5.5	10.0	3.8
	3.5-7.5	6.2-13.8	1.7-5.9

*) One significant difference between durations

**) Two significant differences between durations

16.4 DISCUSSION

The three sub-samples with different durations for states gave the same type of results. The mean values of the health states did not differ significantly from each other between the sub-samples. This similarity was not expected to be as strong as it was found to be. In the convenience sample the duration had systematic effects on the state values. This result was analogous to the earlier studies with the time trade-off method. However, there are no earlier studies with the CR method concerning the effects of the chosen duration on the values assigned to the states.

According to the Finnish EuroQol survey duration is not of great importance when respondents value health states with the CR method. One reason may be that subjects forget the existence of the defined duration in the valuation task when a postal questionnaire is used. Another explanation may be that the cognitive process behind the valuation does not include duration as an important factor. The third possibility is that the CR method does not produce values on an interval scale (see Nord, 1992). If respondents use the CR scale basically for ranking health states then duration would not affect the values of the states. The states simply have a similar ranking with different durations.

When the Finnish EuroQol survey results are examined alongside the convenience sample, the first explanation is most likely - the respondents just forget the existence of time. This means that if we would like to have values for a given duration we should change the standard EuroQol questionnaire in a way that duration is more clearly integrated into the valuation. However, we have first to answer the question: do we need the information about the 'time preference' in the CR method? If a respondent forgets the duration we obtain 'general values' which are, at least partly, 'time indifferent'.

Although it was not possible to find any significant differences between the three EuroQol sub-samples, the 'one year' data proved to be slightly better than the 'ten years' and 'unspecified' data. The response rate and the rate of consistent responses were a little better in the 'one year' sample than in the other two samples. The one year duration seems to be easier for respondents. This may suggest that there is no reason to change the one year duration in the standard EuroQol valuation questionnaire.

One critical question for the Euroqol Group is why so many elderly people did not understand the valuation task. This problem will be discussed further when all the data are analyzed. It may be that we should use interviews at least among the older age groups. In addition a short verbal introduction before the valuation task has proved to be useful (Ohinmaa, 1993).

Presented at the EuroQol Plenary Meeting: Rotterdam, The Netherlands, 1993

16.5 REFERENCES

EuroQol Group. EuroQol - A new facility for the measurement of health related quality of life. Health Policy 1990;16:199-208.

Nord E. Methods for quality adjustment of life years. Social Science and Medicine, 1992;34(5):559-569.

Ohinmaa A. QALYs - Valuation of the EuroQol-measure in different subgroups of Finnish population. Licentiate thesis, University of Oulu, Department of Economics, 1993.

Rosser R, Sintonen H. The EuroQol Quality of Life Project, In: Walker S, Rosser R, editors. Quality of Life Assessment: Key issues in the 1990s. 1993:197-200.

APPENDIX 16.1
The standard EuroQol questionnaire page 4.

- We now want you to consider some other health states.

- Remember, we want you to indicate how good or bad each of these states would be for a person like you.

- They are described, on either side of the scale, on the page opposite.

- When thinking about each health state imagine that it will last for one year. What happens after that is not known and should not be taken into account.

- Please draw **one line from each box** to whichever point on the scale indicates how good or bad the state described in that box is.

- It does not matter if your lines cross each other.

APPENDIX 16.1
The standard EuroQol questionnaire page 5.

Best imaginable health state

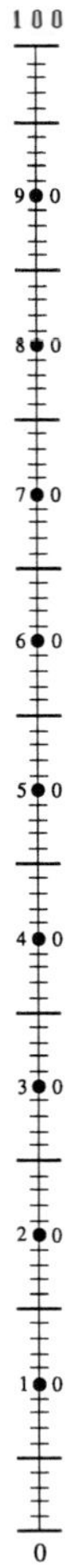

Worst imaginable health state

No problems in walking about
No problems with self-care
Some problems with performing usual activities *(e.g. work, study, housework, family or leisure activities)*
No pain or discomfort
Not anxious or depressed

No problems in walking about
No problems with self-care
No problems with performing usual activities *(e.g. work, study, housework, family or leisure activities)*
Moderate pain or discomfort
Not anxious or depressed

No problems in walking about
No problems with self-care
No problems with performing usual activities *(e.g. work, study, housework, family or leisure activities)*
No pain or discomfort
Not anxious or depressed

Some problems in walking about
Some problems with washing or dressing self
Some problems with performing usual activities *(e.g. work, study, housework, family or leisure activities)*
Extreme pain or discomfort
Extremely anxious or depressed

Some problems in walking about
No problems with self-care
Some problems with performing usual activities *(e.g. work, study, housework, family or leisure activities)*
Extreme pain or discomfort
Moderately anxious or depressed

Confined to bed
Unable to wash or dress self
Unable to perform usual activities *(e.g. work, study, housework, family or leisure activities)*
Extreme pain or discomfort
Extremely anxious or depressed

No problems in walking about
No problems with self-care
No problems with performing usual activities *(e.g. work, study, housework, family or leisure activities)*
Moderate pain or discomfort
Moderately anxious or depressed

Confined to bed
Unable to wash or dress self
Unable to perform usual activities *(e.g. work, study, housework, family or leisure activities)*
Moderate pain or discomfort
Not anxious or depressed

PLEASE CHECK THAT YOU HAVE DRAWN ONE LINE FROM EACH BOX (THAT IS, 8 LINES IN ALL)

APPENDIX 16.1
The standard EuroQol questionnaire page 6.

IN THE SAME WAY AS ON THE PREVIOUS PAGE, PLEASE INDICATE HOW GOOD OR BAD THESE ADDITIONAL STATES ARE, BY DRAWING A LINE FROM EACH BOX TO A POINT ON THE SCALE.

YOU WILL FIND THAT 2 OF THESE STATES (MARKED *) ARE REPEATED FROM THE PREVIOUS PAGE.

Best imaginable health state

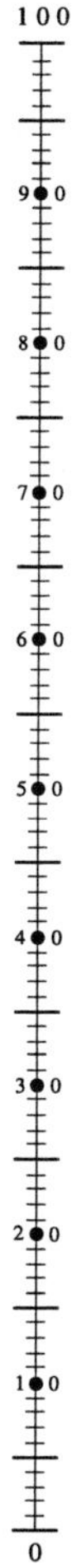

Worst imaginable health state

Some problems in walking about
No problems with self-care
No problems with performing usual activities *(e.g. work, study, housework, family or leisure activities)*
No pain or discomfort
Not anxious or depressed

No problems in walking about
No problems with self-care
No problems with performing usual activities *(e.g. work, study, housework, family or leisure activities)*
No pain or discomfort
Moderately anxious or depressed

No problems in walking about *
No problems with self-care
No problems with performing usual activities *(e.g. work, study, housework, family or leisure activities)*
No pain or discomfort
Not anxious or depressed

Confined to bed
Some problems with washing or dressing self
Some problems with performing usual activities *(e.g. work, study, housework, family or leisure activities)*
No pain or discomfort
Not anxious or depressed

Unconscious

Confined to bed *
Unable to wash or dress self
Unable to perform usual activities *(e.g. work, study, housework, family or leisure activities)*
Extreme pain or discomfort
Extremely anxious or depressed

No problems in walking about
Some problems with washing or dressing self
No problems with performing usual activities *(e.g. work, study, housework, family or leisure activities)*
No pain or discomfort
Not anxious or depressed

Some problems in walking about
Some problems with washing or dressing self
Unable to perform usual activities *(e.g. work, study, housework, family or leisure activities)*
Moderate pain or discomfort
Extremely anxious or depressed

PLEASE CHECK THAT YOU HAVE DRAWN ONE LINE FROM EACH BOX (THAT IS, 8 LINES IN ALL)

17
Applying paired comparisons models to EQ-5D valuations - deriving TTO utilities from ordinal preference data

Paul Kind

17.1 BACKGROUND

The use of paired comparisons methods as a means of eliciting valuations for health states was first proposed by Fanshel and Bush in their seminal 1970 paper (Fanshel and Bush, 1970). However, it has seldom been applied in this role, a notable exception being the Nottingham Health Profile (McKenna, 1981). Given its simplicity and the low demands it makes of respondents, it is perhaps surprising that it has not found wider acceptance. Were such a low-cost technique found to adequately represent valuations obtained through more sophisticated means, then this might open the door to more widespread investigation of health state values in population studies or in clinical sub-groups, particularly where large numbers of participants might push up the costs of collecting such data. The results presented here represent an empirical investigation of the relationship between valuations produced directly using a TTO procedure, and scale values arising from the application of paired comparisons models to ordinal preference data generated by participants in the 1993 MVH survey of the UK population. Since that survey probably represents the largest study of its kind, the data set generated by it should prove sufficient to adequately test the power of paired comparisons modeling.

Paired comparisons methods had been in widespread use in the investigation of physical sensation for some time before Thurstone first published his Law of Comparative Judgement (Thurstone, 1927). In a typical experimental situation, subjects are repeatedly required to choose between two physical stimuli of varying magnitudes. Such stimuli might be light, weight or sound. Given a standard stimulus (say a light of fixed intensity), a subject would be asked to compare it with a second stimulus, and to indicate which of the two was greater. In classical psychophysics, the investigator might vary the magnitude of the second stimulus until the subject was unable to detect a difference between the two stimuli - a so-called jnd (just-noticeable-difference). In such confusion methods, the probability of a subject indicating that one stimulus is greater than the other is seen as functionally related to the difference between the pair in terms of their physical magnitude. If the two stimuli are of equal intensity, then the probability of either being designated as greater than its pair will be equal (p = 0.5). The probability that the more intense stimulus will be so chosen will be greater than 0.5 (and similarly, that the lower intensity stimulus will be chosen

P. Kind et al. (eds.), EQ-5D concepts and methods, 201–220.

has a probability of less than 0.5). Where there is no confusion and one stimulus always dominates the other, then probabilities are 1 and 0 respectively.

During the late 1920s the work of Thurstone extended this general approach to a representation of judgements made in regard to non-physical continua such as the seriousness of crime (Thurstone, 1928). In his model, the separation of stimuli is represented on an underlying single-dimensioned psychological continuum on which the distances between pairs of stimuli is a function of the probability of one stimulus being selected as having a degree of intensity greater than that of its pair. Although psychologists typically refer to stimuli, in the present context it will be more natural to refer to health states, and to characterise the underlying psychological attribute as 'severity'.

Thurstone's law of comparative judgement (Thurstone, 1927) is based on the concept that the assessment of any stimulus (in this case health states) with respect to a specific attribute (severity) can be represented by a theoretical distribution of points located along an underlying psychological continuum. This distribution is termed the discriminal process, and is assumed to be normal. The scale value of a state is given by the the mean of the discriminal process.

In general, if a subject is asked to make repeated judgements, a state will sometimes be regarded as more, and sometimes as less severe, than any other state with which it is compared. When s/he makes a single judgement about which of the two states has the greater severity, it is assumed that s/he samples from the separate distributions which individually characterise each state. Given two health states, X and Y, then when judgements about their relative severity are made, the severity of each state is drawn from its corresponding hypothesised distribution (as shown in Figure 17.1).

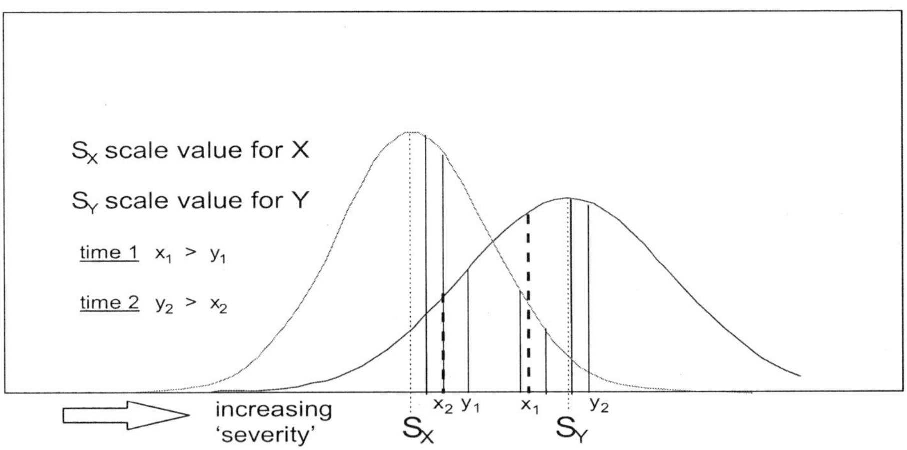

Figure 17.1 Graphical representation of classical Thurstone model

In this example the first comparison of states X and Y are represented by x_1 and y_2, corresponding to a judgement that Y > X. Similarly x_2 and y_2 represent a second comparison between the states in which X >Y.

Thurstone postulated a model (the Law of Comparative Judgement) based on the mechanisms described above, which produced a theoretical framework that could be used to estimate scale values for subjective continua - such as health state severity. The full model is given by the following equation

$$v_x - v_y = z_{xy} \cdot (\sigma_x^2 + \sigma_y^2 - 2r_{xy} \cdot \sigma_x \cdot \sigma_y)^{1/2} \tag{17.1}$$

Where $v_x - v_y$ is the difference in scale values for states X and Y (i.e. the difference in means of the two discriminal dispersions associated with X and Y)

z_{xy} is the normal deviate corresponding to the proportion of times that state X is judged more severe than state Y

σ_x and σ_y are the standard deviations of the discriminal dispersions of states X and Y

r_{xy} is the correlation between the two discriminal dispersions

Thurstone further postulated a number of simplifying assumptions (Cases I to V) under which it is possible to solve the full model - for example that all σ are equal, as are intercorrelations between discriminal dispersions. Under these assumptions (Case V), the residual term $[\sigma^2 . (1 - r)]^{1/2}$ becomes a constant and defines the unit of measurement of the severity scale on which health states are located.

The computational steps involved in deriving scale values are quite straightforward. Firstly, a frequency matrix F_{ij} is constructed, in which the ij^{th} element indicates the number of occasions on which state i is judged to be more severe than state j. The leading diagonal element (F_{ij}) is set to zero since no state is compared with itself. The frequencies held in the F-matrix are then converted into a corresponding P-matrix containing proportions where $P_{ij} = F_{ij} / (F_{ij} + F_{ji})$. Finally, the P-matrix is converted to unit normal values (z-scores), corresponding to their location on a normal distribution with a mean of 0 and a standard deviation of 1. Extreme values of p (equal to 1 or 0) and arising from near certain preferences, are flagged as missing values since the equivalent z-scores would be infinity. Scale values for each state are given by the mean value of the column total, calculated using all non-missing elements in the Z-matrix. A goodness-of-fit statistic can calculated by reversing the computational process. Taking the computed scores for each state, it is possible to calculate the expected difference between all pairs of states - representing differences in terms of their z-scores. These values can be back-transformed to determine the expected probability that one state will be judged to be more severe than another. The difference between these expected probabilities and those observed in the raw data can be computed for all pairs of states and yields an average discrepancy - used as a goodness-of-fit statistic, and which (according to Edwards, 1957) is of the order of 0.05 for most paired comparisons studies where the model adequately fits the data.

17.2 DATA

This paper reports on the use of paired comparisons models in the analysis of two datasets. The first of these consists of the ordinal preferences contained within the TTO values recorded by 2997 respondents who took part in the national UK survey conducted by the MVH Group in 1993.

These data and the survey methods used to generate them, have been previously reported and will not be rehearsed again here. In the present paper, however, it is not the values themselves which are subject to analysis, but rather the ordinal relationship between states that is implied by the values they are given. For a given subject, with a fixed set of health states, a state which receives a value of 0.8 is preferred to all states which attract a lower value. Hence by comparing all pairs of states directly valued by all individuals in the MVH survey, it is possible to construct an F-matrix that records their aggregate pairwise preferences.

The second data set consists of ordinal preferences expressed more simply. As an initial familiarisation task, the MVH protocol required individuals to rank order all the states which they were subsequently asked to value. Inspection of the ranking generated by each individual enabled a second F-matrix to be constructed, but in this instance the relationships are not inferred from the relative values, but can be taken directly from the observed ranking of states. A state ranked 5th, for example, is taken as preferred to all other states ranked below it.

The state 11111 (no problem on any of the 5 EuroQol dimensions) and by definition the logically 'best' state within the TTO procedure, has a predetermined position as the most preferred health state, and as such cannot be included in a paired comparisons model since its ordinal relationship with other states is never 'confused' - an essential requirement of the Thurstone model. Similarly, in ranking states, individuals always placed 11111 as the highest (best possible) health state. The ordinal relationship between all other states (including unconscious and death) could be determined by inspecting respondents' TTO valuations. Reinterpreting the TTO data in this way produces a 44 x 44 frequency matrix that contains the number of occasions that each state was 'preferred' to every other state.

Table 17.1 presents the full F-matrix constructed using the implied preferences in the TTO data generated by 2997 respondents. It will be seen that 255 respondents consider that state 1 (32211) dominates state 4 (11112) (row 1 column 4), whereas only 13 respondents hold the contrary view (row 4 column 1). It will be apparent from Table 17.1 that not all states were valued on an equal number of occasions. In some instances, the judgement as to which state dominates its pair is almost equally divided, for example for states 18 and 19, 32331 and 12223 each respectively recording 75 and 76 'votes' in favour. The corresponding F-matrix derived from the preferences expressed in the ranking task are given in Table 17.2.

Tables 17.3 and 17.4 presents extracts from the P-matrices corresponding to the frequencies shown in Table 17.1 and 17.2. The probability of selecting 32211 as more severe than 11112 is 0.951 as judged in terms of the TTO preferences in Table 17.1, and the equivalent probability in Table 17.2 is 0.976. It will be noted that not all probabilities are as similar in the two matrices, for example in comparing 32211 with death the probabilites become 0.355 and 0.094 respectively.

Table 17.5 shows the scale values from the Thurstone model as applied to the TTO preference data. The average discrepancy for this model was computed to be 0.03. The scale values range from 1.823 to -1.744 and as with such models, sum to 0. On this basis, the state 21111 is ranked as the least severe state, and so as to make these 'raw' scale values comparable with the mean observed TTO values which lie on a conventional 0-1 scale, the Thurstone values were transformed as follows

$$TTO_{est} = K \,.\, [Th_i - Th_{dead}] \,/\, [Th_{21111} - Th_{dead}] \qquad (17.2)$$

where K = 0.878 (the mean observed TTO score for the state 21111) and Th_i, Th_{21111} and Th_{dead} are the Thurstone scale values for the ith states and for states 21111 and dead respectively, and TTO_{est} is the estimated value recovered from the Thurstone scale values.

The mean difference between the transformed Thurstone scale values and the directly observed TTO means is 0.006.

Table 17.6 gives the corresponding scale values computed from the preference data extracted from the ranking task. The results from the Thurstone model have in this instance been standardised using a value for K of 0.850, since in this model the state 11121 received the highest value, and K is set to the equivalent value of the mean observed TTO for that state.

Table 17.1 Implied preferences from TTO valuations

	32211	23321	11211	11112	death	12121	21232	13332	12222	12211	33212	21312	33323	33232	11113	22323	32223	32331	12223	11131	32232	11133
32211	0	70	266	255	252	161	59	32	75	151	39	112	17	23	113	57	24	5	61	74	26	58
23321	101	0	274	265	264	200	82	18	147	161	29	128	15	17	109	38	20	24	84	89	25	51
11211	7	7	0	85	6	26	5	1	24	47	5	25	0	2	19	8	3	0	14	8	2	6
11112	13	9	99	0	24	60	10	4	25	70	9	31	5	3	23	5	3	4	17	16	5	7
death	457	455	1197	1172	0	742	411	230	642	724	362	622	138	167	564	386	260	198	484	458	230	344
12121	11	8	166	151	20	0	6	2	35	45	6	17	5	2	19	5	3	5	16	10	6	8
21232	69	90	288	301	315	178	0	31	121	176	72	150	38	20	128	84	41	23	62	90	40	55
13332	130	113	282	281	461	178	129	0	169	168	82	172	31	35	133	73	57	56	154	126	64	91
12222	27	26	215	197	79	120	11	11	0	121	14	69	3	5	49	17	6	7	24	35	8	22
12211	9	7	133	127	20	41	5	1	22	0	6	26	3	4	18	4	4	1	13	9	1	9
33212	123	67	299	283	363	164	104	43	154	175	0	146	14	20	134	61	31	37	116	109	41	77
21312	37	28	214	181	80	92	20	4	81	82	4	0	4	5	44	16	13	6	33	31	9	26
33323	157	92	315	290	587	204	130	75	164	181	107	190	0	53	162	113	86	95	163	136	67	124
33232	144	117	298	312	539	195	146	74	191	180	92	174	48	0	190	106	76	78	154	156	87	102
11113	61	47	210	224	149	86	53	21	93	92	38	69	9	17	0	36	19	21	41	47	24	15
22323	101	68	281	265	317	177	80	23	132	188	56	136	21	19	116	0	31	48	99	91	38	71
32223	139	92	282	281	445	169	94	55	176	178	87	166	32	28	160	78	0	51	140	123	55	76
32331	110	144	288	270	493	190	96	91	134	177	123	170	60	53	155	134	77	0	95	145	95	109
12223	60	82	293	273	234	159	38	33	107	147	62	124	15	16	104	47	25	20	0	75	28	41
11131	88	82	241	277	246	101	63	20	121	105	65	85	26	17	84	67	45	28	76	0	27	26
32232	129	99	267	269	483	176	103	53	146	166	77	163	23	35	140	70	48	56	138	132	0	97
11133	123	112	294	284	374	132	112	55	148	135	100	109	42	31	100	84	72	53	114	80	46	0
33321	112	92	291	278	415	167	116	51	188	152	76	144	23	30	142	67	49	41	118	111	48	102
22331	83	96	264	246	345	163	72	45	102	174	81	147	33	30	125	83	53	26	85	103	54	73
13311	37	40	243	246	165	145	31	25	90	144	31	96	11	15	88	33	20	15	42	49	20	50
21323	64	86	261	272	246	141	47	31	98	164	55	128	16	20	104	58	38	20	63	100	29	47
12111	9	3	87	87	22	40	6	0	18	51	5	26	4	3	21	9	4	6	19	18	2	14
13212	36	37	258	239	145	136	33	9	88	146	29	100	6	8	87	32	12	5	40	63	18	25
22233	127	88	303	306	420	176	141	46	163	174	71	168	38	35	165	86	52	58	142	131	56	115
32313	91	106	295	279	430	188	87	65	108	172	89	156	29	48	166	112	73	35	109	112	64	85
22222	33	39	232	233	97	142	22	9	56	152	24	71	2	8	68	27	14	6	37	42	16	21
22112	23	13	212	189	36	66	14	5	38	78	8	33	3	2	37	3	7	8	20	18	4	6
11121	13	11	89	83	12	55	5	2	15	59	7	24	1	1	29	4	3	1	8	10	3	4
22121	19	12	201	187	51	72	10	5	51	81	13	33	4	3	30	9	10	0	23	22	6	7
uncon	597	581	1196	1189	2432	762	567	425	703	736	541	682	309	355	652	542	459	388	611	565	409	485
22122	28	20	220	222	79	123	16	5	52	117	12	61	5	3	67	13	8	6	20	38	7	26
21111	5	7	74	71	10	25	2	1	13	44	1	18	1	3	15	2	3	2	5	11	2	7
21222	28	33	229	210	75	92	16	6	49	90	17	42	8	2	39	15	5	2	34	26	4	8
23313	124	74	266	279	369	169	110	39	154	172	58	151	22	30	148	54	42	59	117	99	26	76
33333	663	660	1194	1193	2573	758	655	558	721	735	621	694	463	485	702	632	562	506	680	657	551	603
21133	113	122	303	261	379	140	96	63	166	103	87	111	31	36	104	83	68	45	117	95	56	60
23232	104	86	281	275	367	167	102	38	152	184	62	143	22	25	119	69	44	40	113	119	46	82
11312	39	28	227	211	80	88	21	8	83	75	13	55	5	8	45	16	12	10	39	20	11	11
11122	13	15	180	166	0	56	9	5	28	49	14	17	2	3	18	11	5	4	9	16	7	5

Table 17.1 Implied preferences from TTO valuations (continued)

33321	22331	13311	21323	12111	13212	22233	32313	22222	22112	11121	22121	uncon	22122	21111	21222	23313	33333	21133	23232	11312	11122	
29	31	74	52	265	77	47	23	99	140	267	149	88	101	271	133	48	35	47	41	139	132	32211
32	52	104	70	275	135	36	27	116	174	257	146	110	146	269	121	29	36	49	38	125	148	23321
1	8	7	8	76	15	3	2	23	28	82	34	7	29	85	22	4	4	5	4	26	45	11211
10	7	18	10	94	19	2	5	21	32	101	40	6	26	108	36	7	4	3	7	32	42	11112
279	358	554	462	1162	585	288	272	647	714	1182	702	111	651	1162	656	336	187	326	305	645	697	death
10	4	25	8	183	17	4	4	25	38	165	28	4	24	165	22	7	4	2	3	26	32	12121
56	35	91	58	268	100	43	41	103	178	277	176	135	114	270	133	62	47	51	40	145	153	21232
60	102	143	119	279	153	59	81	159	180	284	190	224	168	287	154	74	86	106	65	174	145	13332
16	15	35	13	227	33	11	5	42	110	228	113	27	50	219	73	14	12	12	12	71	98	12222
5	4	16	8	132	13	0	3	23	23	137	27	6	30	150	21	5	5	6	2	17	44	12211
40	78	140	123	278	131	47	49	147	177	289	170	162	148	278	163	59	70	82	52	139	166	33212
13	16	49	21	217	53	8	10	67	68	232	61	30	77	213	51	17	8	12	11	48	69	21312
83	138	164	141	278	185	84	122	191	168	311	201	321	176	287	163	113	133	134	90	183	164	33323
72	124	182	136	298	160	92	124	187	162	294	197	281	170	272	165	82	119	108	83	177	183	33232
32	34	77	42	233	71	13	21	98	94	244	82	66	96	240	65	28	22	19	27	72	86	11113
49	73	116	93	269	152	35	40	140	163	272	166	148	154	278	162	48	51	68	43	153	154	22323
61	99	149	135	279	162	50	76	170	173	297	155	215	163	285	165	72	77	88	53	151	176	32223
77	70	97	98	293	119	105	72	131	179	301	167	260	105	261	155	115	100	98	78	143	150	32331
40	29	79	48	257	80	27	16	99	162	254	153	101	97	242	125	34	34	39	37	119	166	12223
54	46	86	78	233	121	34	39	116	101	260	104	127	114	237	78	62	35	27	36	87	103	11131
60	99	144	130	310	162	49	79	171	181	281	170	234	171	292	168	73	83	90	74	158	182	32232
71	79	118	113	267	133	50	63	154	112	268	109	197	144	275	118	88	68	47	67	105	120	11133
0	104	152	124	294	152	58	80	151	189	279	143	205	148	268	164	76	85	88	53	169	171	33321
58	0	88	91	272	110	46	44	101	149	282	167	176	106	293	155	84	61	60	63	151	170	22331
22	21	0	34	233	62	26	16	78	130	248	118	64	74	254	98	16	24	37	21	103	123	13311
60	51	78	0	259	86	24	26	85	145	265	141	102	103	265	162	49	41	53	42	131	147	21323
3	9	14	15	0	7	2	4	16	23	85	28	8	28	96	28	3	4	5	5	31	39	12111
20	20	48	21	251	0	15	20	69	120	240	130	52	67	244	111	19	21	22	24	99	123	13212
60	93	146	99	275	146	0	80	183	181	279	184	216	166	290	165	84	80	95	61	152	174	22233
78	76	108	79	289	106	87	0	133	165	297	189	202	126	277	189	95	81	99	110	158	168	32313
16	14	52	24	268	40	10	8	0	108	249	103	33	68	221	74	18	17	18	11	81	157	22222
9	10	27	14	187	38	9	11	34	0	198	49	8	53	198	39	7	4	6	8	32	63	22112
4	3	25	1	77	16	2	7	20	40	0	30	4	19	110	22	4	4	4	4	26	42	11121
11	8	31	22	212	37	7	7	40	60	201	0	20	42	199	39	10	4	12	7	47	55	22121
452	500	642	601	1178	664	474	459	717	746	1193	733	0	701	1162	689	498	740	490	469	698	715	uncon
16	7	33	19	189	44	5	4	39	87	204	89	25	0	244	76	11	12	15	9	75	100	22122
3	6	10	3	67	9	1	4	13	26	56	19	7	16	0	13	2	4	3	0	23	45	21111
16	12	49	14	200	63	14	6	58	55	217	61	29	58	227	0	13	8	8	9	56	82	21222
41	63	133	108	290	137	45	49	159	170	297	164	176	179	281	155	0	49	69	37	174	163	23313
564	603	685	665	1170	694	580	571	735	743	1194	743	1708	713	1157	717	615	0	612	574	716	718	33333
76	75	154	106	289	136	54	62	156	122	263	120	184	166	285	108	76	54	0	67	122	116	21133
41	78	138	109	267	150	30	81	168	163	279	173	182	160	266	160	58	71	68	0	159	164	23232
14	19	60	28	197	50	11	9	74	64	221	57	29	82	220	64	14	13	10	9	0	85	11312
6	16	30	15	156	18	4	8	30	28	137	37	14	41	174	32	9	8	6	4	28	0	11122

Table 17.2 Preferences extracted from ranking task

	32211	23321	11211	11112	death	12121	21232	13332	12222	12211	33212	21312	33323	33232	11113	22323	32223	32331	12223	11131	32232	11133
32211	0	99	292	283	70	187	87	58	113	179	23	153	5	8	158	82	22	4	92	121	14	99
23321	93	0	296	287	59	220	121	26	184	181	31	164	4	11	155	52	24	12	136	134	18	95
11211	5	8	0	159	6	20	3	2	14	16	3	6	5	4	36	3	3	2	7	10	0	2
11112	7	6	129	0	10	44	5	2	7	69	1	5	1	1	10	1	2	2	6	14	1	7
death	674	685	1200	1192	0	764	700	611	735	743	660	701	519	562	714	652	602	576	710	676	600	678
12121	7	2	271	264	5	0	8	2	15	82	1	13	3	2	36	2	1	1	8	12	0	5
21232	55	76	304	321	56	184	0	17	131	184	45	141	13	10	160	51	23	5	70	159	16	72
13332	122	111	290	291	118	183	171	0	181	175	84	177	19	32	153	83	52	69	189	157	73	143
12222	7	7	291	280	11	180	11	3	0	175	6	35	1	2	68	6	3	4	7	45	2	15
12211	3	2	261	237	5	47	8	2	15	0	0	8	1	1	32	2	1	2	2	13	2	5
33212	159	77	313	309	98	183	147	52	179	191	0	157	4	11	167	89	43	38	161	145	52	118
21312	16	11	279	257	22	120	43	5	149	130	8	0	2	4	78	11	9	6	53	56	7	27
33323	182	116	319	295	232	208	176	110	168	189	139	199	0	86	175	142	125	146	184	159	93	166
33232	174	141	304	321	184	198	179	104	205	189	114	180	30	0	204	119	104	128	168	185	123	140
11113	35	27	247	292	37	98	39	19	103	104	29	58	6	13	0	7	6	14	27	49	13	11
22323	95	76	303	290	87	190	129	31	163	207	45	164	7	15	167	0	21	32	149	133	31	120
32223	163	107	292	291	135	175	132	77	193	191	85	182	9	22	189	100	0	59	172	164	65	118
32331	121	178	301	282	153	201	132	109	142	183	144	183	38	33	173	164	97	0	117	184	131	164
12223	41	56	323	304	42	183	46	18	130	171	45	128	3	9	149	17	11	12	0	108	24	32
11131	55	55	267	309	53	114	22	8	131	108	49	69	12	5	80	39	25	8	72	0	7	7
32232	159	114	279	286	144	193	155	67	161	169	94	171	17	11	169	93	59	46	161	182	0	138
11133	92	87	310	302	75	146	121	43	171	149	81	117	25	20	120	58	49	33	138	121	45	0
33321	152	129	302	296	136	183	170	84	205	164	112	162	13	28	167	95	88	56	160	145	82	153
22331	71	106	278	270	96	177	103	34	127	191	77	174	15	10	153	80	46	9	91	152	43	107
13311	45	30	280	296	33	187	56	11	132	182	26	133	5	7	136	45	26	10	83	89	28	66
21323	61	85	287	304	64	164	80	33	126	187	62	149	10	12	158	42	33	17	107	142	42	90
12111	5	2	172	172	4	26	7	2	9	22	1	11	1	2	34	4	5	3	9	18	2	9
13212	29	23	296	293	37	173	40	14	119	169	10	91	4	5	130	28	7	8	42	114	12	35
22233	114	104	313	318	110	192	181	43	181	183	74	170	20	38	180	89	44	56	184	162	45	155
32313	120	134	302	295	118	199	130	116	116	182	119	165	11	43	192	139	109	45	138	149	93	147
22222	12	15	298	300	17	190	23	10	102	190	14	66	4	3	75	8	3	3	35	54	8	26
22112	5	10	302	280	12	112	18	8	59	106	5	23	3	0	64	6	5	1	30	23	1	16
11121	4	1	143	136	6	15	4	2	6	55	2	9	2	2	22	0	1	2	4	10	1	4
22121	7	3	289	284	9	106	14	8	61	125	1	18	2	0	39	4	2	2	20	29	2	9
uncon	683	683	1198	1191	966	762	699	616	732	742	671	700	536	577	712	667	625	593	715	664	618	681
22122	12	12	286	303	12	157	14	11	67	165	7	44	3	0	72	3	2	2	17	48	9	21
21111	4	6	141	151	8	46	3	4	22	43	0	5	2	1	37	3	0	0	12	15	0	7
21222	12	10	294	294	20	122	15	5	83	135	4	27	5	3	40	9	2	2	21	38	4	13
23313	130	88	278	294	101	183	145	51	190	189	76	171	12	23	174	75	50	51	151	145	53	125
33333	729	737	1203	1197	1305	767	759	721	746	747	744	722	706	716	745	729	728	712	750	726	729	747
21133	104	90	322	279	91	152	127	45	183	116	79	114	24	34	122	63	59	27	149	132	55	103
23232	105	100	292	292	81	172	153	28	176	193	58	154	17	10	143	83	38	23	146	151	37	112
11312	30	15	283	284	26	121	18	3	134	112	5	27	3	3	65	7	6	2	38	33	5	9
11122	6	6	262	265	6	50	1	2	9	63	5	5	1	0	11	1	3	2	8	11	1	5

Table 17.2 Preferences extracted from ranking task (continued)

	33321	22331	13311	21323	12111	13212	22233	32313	22222	22112	11121	22121	uncon	22122	21111	21222	23313	33333	21133	23232	11312	11122
32211	9	54	80	72	297	96	77	14	138	176	301	183	59	132	288	174	69	8	78	63	165	157
23321	10	53	143	90	298	164	36	19	163	186	294	177	62	174	291	166	30	6	94	39	151	168
11211	2	3	6	4	89	7	2	3	8	15	130	14	8	15	113	12	2	5	7	3	18	49
11112	4	5	5	7	98	3	2	1	8	14	150	22	11	8	123	7	3	4	1	2	9	23
death	602	641	704	680	1187	706	646	634	749	746	1196	751	1730	727	1168	717	645	1534	657	640	719	729
12121	3	2	6	3	275	16	2	1	10	25	297	24	6	23	242	19	3	3	2	2	21	71
21232	26	23	79	38	288	100	23	23	114	186	299	190	57	124	285	157	40	1	41	20	155	171
13332	39	135	163	146	285	153	79	59	171	186	295	193	107	167	293	169	77	9	150	93	187	160
12222	6	4	15	4	286	20	3	2	20	130	294	132	12	57	277	71	6	1	10	4	44	157
12211	3	1	6	2	268	6	2	2	10	14	237	24	5	15	249	8	0	0	2	2	13	63
33212	23	107	153	146	293	167	65	43	168	190	309	194	88	177	292	195	58	9	113	73	166	190
21312	5	7	34	20	288	80	17	3	110	101	294	99	23	126	282	92	9	1	16	9	108	114
33323	120	179	179	167	288	192	118	170	200	171	312	211	209	183	294	174	140	21	170	121	189	171
33232	89	162	197	163	303	173	108	152	199	169	296	204	158	181	280	171	114	17	147	122	188	194
11113	19	21	54	17	265	46	9	8	109	100	297	96	38	119	251	81	13	6	11	26	64	108
22323	33	100	131	131	292	180	50	41	172	176	291	183	71	178	294	182	42	7	104	46	178	174
32223	57	131	163	158	285	176	73	69	188	181	309	172	112	180	298	188	81	6	130	82	169	185
32331	79	111	116	121	302	122	137	76	146	198	312	175	133	120	271	174	144	9	147	117	161	160
12223	16	41	60	28	293	95	7	2	112	174	286	177	38	117	262	168	15	2	27	23	133	198
11131	32	17	71	49	262	94	17	17	124	111	288	107	64	127	258	78	29	2	14	19	85	127
32232	43	145	150	143	325	172	73	83	189	195	290	184	118	181	309	177	63	7	122	109	181	201
11133	49	79	101	95	288	133	32	32	171	111	287	115	70	166	290	126	62	5	22	67	118	126
33321	0	145	176	162	305	176	91	108	170	201	288	160	115	165	280	182	95	14	146	70	189	185
22331	42	0	82	95	298	117	49	30	124	163	292	184	88	121	319	179	62	5	83	78	173	193
13311	13	34	0	45	276	93	35	11	110	160	300	159	41	113	284	132	19	9	60	36	163	163
21323	37	56	82	0	287	95	34	11	113	172	284	165	63	132	294	200	36	4	76	45	174	179
12111	0	3	7	9	0	8	2	1	8	9	172	14	9	14	160	20	1	3	5	1	25	58
13212	4	20	36	28	284	0	20	3	90	160	275	162	36	92	292	150	12	1	31	12	123	160
22233	43	125	156	109	285	152	0	66	203	193	295	194	104	176	299	186	74	15	144	60	167	191
32313	76	115	116	109	308	129	126	0	146	180	313	201	103	135	287	200	122	11	152	157	181	184
22222	7	6	37	15	310	42	6	3	0	159	310	155	12	103	274	146	7	2	17	3	87	216
22112	2	5	26	14	270	23	2	1	16	0	288	62	9	28	288	35	4	3	4	3	26	108
11121	1	3	10	7	102	13	2	1	7	23	0	8	7	10	141	8	2	3	4	2	18	21
22121	1	5	25	15	296	27	2	1	16	80	298	0	10	30	264	37	8	1	13	2	33	104
uncon	621	645	693	680	1181	706	652	644	754	750	1195	750	0	725	1161	719	655	1592	665	636	724	720
22122	8	3	17	11	254	37	7	1	21	147	264	130	15	0	305	78	5	4	7	5	73	170
21111	2	2	11	4	127	8	2	2	7	14	133	21	15	9	0	10	2	3	5	0	23	71
21222	9	9	30	6	269	49	3	7	20	87	277	84	19	77	276	0	5	4	7	0	45	134
23313	34	97	148	156	306	161	77	43	181	184	313	179	88	202	294	174	0	8	107	54	202	184
33333	713	730	728	741	1189	740	739	734	762	756	1200	759	1249	736	1174	734	730	0	740	714	747	732
21133	44	83	145	111	304	136	36	44	172	133	271	126	85	190	298	120	62	5	0	67	122	124
23232	42	96	136	125	285	167	44	54	194	188	293	190	83	171	278	182	56	7	106	0	173	174
11312	6	11	31	12	273	53	10	1	107	98	287	102	22	121	272	105	9	1	16	5	0	0
11122	2	5	12	6	218	8	0	2	9	19	249	27	13	12	232	8	1	2	4	3	0	0

Table 17.3 Upper segment of probability matrix corresponding to F-matrix based on TTO valuations

	32211	23321	11211	11112	death	12121	21232	13332	12222	12211	33212	21312	33323
32211	0	0.409	0.974	0.951	0.355	0.936	0.461	0.198	0.735	0.944	0.241	0.752	0.098
23321	0.591	0	0.975	0.967	0.367	0.962	0.477	0.137	0.850	0.958	0.302	0.821	0.140
11211	0.026	0.025	0	0.462	0.005	0.135	0.017	0.004	0.100	0.261	0.016	0.105	0.000
11112	0.049	0.033	0.538	0	0.020	0.284	0.032	0.014	0.113	0.355	0.031	0.146	0.017
death	0.645	0.633	0.995	0.980	0	0.974	0.566	0.333	0.890	0.973	0.499	0.886	0.190
12121	0.064	0.038	0.865	0.716	0.026	0	0.033	0.011	0.226	0.523	0.035	0.156	0.024
21232	0.539	0.523	0.983	0.968	0.434	0.967	0	0.194	0.917	0.972	0.409	0.882	0.226
13332	0.802	0.863	0.996	0.986	0.667	0.989	0.806	0	0.939	0.994	0.656	0.977	0.292
12222	0.265	0.150	0.900	0.887	0.110	0.774	0.083	0.061	0	0.846	0.083	0.460	0.018
12211	0.056	0.042	0.739	0.645	0.027	0.477	0.028	0.006	0.154	0	0.033	0.241	0.016
33212	0.759	0.698	0.984	0.969	0.501	0.965	0.591	0.344	0.917	0.967	0	0.973	0.116
21312	0.248	0.179	0.895	0.854	0.114	0.844	0.118	0.023	0.540	0.759	0.027	0	0.021
33323	0.902	0.860	1.000	0.983	0.810	0.976	0.774	0.708	0.982	0.984	0.884	0.979	0
33232	0.862	0.873	0.993	0.990	0.763	0.990	0.880	0.679	0.974	0.978	0.821	0.972	0.475
11113	0.351	0.301	0.917	0.907	0.209	0.819	0.293	0.136	0.655	0.836	0.221	0.611	0.053
22323	0.639	0.642	0.972	0.981	0.451	0.973	0.488	0.240	0.886	0.979	0.479	0.895	0.157
32223	0.853	0.821	0.989	0.989	0.631	0.983	0.696	0.491	0.967	0.978	0.737	0.927	0.271
32331	0.957	0.857	1.000	0.985	0.713	0.974	0.807	0.619	0.950	0.994	0.769	0.966	0.387
12223	0.496	0.494	0.954	0.941	0.326	0.909	0.380	0.176	0.817	0.919	0.348	0.790	0.084
11131	0.543	0.480	0.968	0.945	0.349	0.910	0.412	0.137	0.776	0.921	0.374	0.733	0.160
32232	0.832	0.798	0.993	0.982	0.677	0.967	0.720	0.453	0.948	0.994	0.653	0.948	0.256
11133	0.680	0.687	0.980	0.976	0.521	0.943	0.671	0.377	0.871	0.938	0.565	0.807	0.253
33321	0.794	0.742	0.997	0.965	0.598	0.944	0.674	0.459	0.922	0.968	0.655	0.917	0.217
22331	0.728	0.649	0.971	0.972	0.491	0.976	0.673	0.306	0.872	0.978	0.509	0.902	0.193
13311	0.333	0.278	0.972	0.932	0.229	0.853	0.254	0.149	0.720	0.900	0.181	0.662	0.063
21323	0.552	0.551	0.970	0.965	0.347	0.946	0.448	0.207	0.883	0.953	0.309	0.859	0.102
12111	0.033	0.011	0.534	0.481	0.019	0.179	0.022	0.000	0.073	0.279	0.018	0.107	0.014
13212	0.319	0.215	0.945	0.926	0.199	0.889	0.248	0.056	0.727	0.918	0.181	0.654	0.031
22233	0.730	0.710	0.990	0.994	0.593	0.978	0.766	0.438	0.937	1.000	0.602	0.955	0.311
32313	0.798	0.797	0.993	0.982	0.613	0.979	0.680	0.445	0.956	0.983	0.645	0.940	0.192

Table 17.4 Upper segment of probability matrix corresponding to F-matrix based on ranking task

	32211	23321	11211	11112	death	12121	21232	13332	12222	12211	33212	21312	33323
32211	0	0.516	0.983	0.976	0.094	0.964	0.613	0.322	0.942	0.984	0.126	0.905	0.027
23321	0.484	0	0.974	0.98	0.079	0.991	0.614	0.19	0.963	0.989	0.287	0.937	0.033
11211	0.017	0.026	0	0.552	0.005	0.069	0.01	0.007	0.046	0.058	0.009	0.021	0.015
11112	0.024	0.02	0.448	0	0.008	0.143	0.015	0.007	0.024	0.225	0.003	0.019	0.003
death	0.906	0.921	0.995	0.992	0	0.993	0.926	0.838	0.985	0.993	0.871	0.97	0.691
12121	0.036	0.009	0.931	0.857	0.007	0	0.042	0.011	0.077	0.636	0.005	0.098	0.014
21232	0.387	0.386	0.99	0.985	0.074	0.958	0	0.09	0.923	0.958	0.234	0.766	0.069
13332	0.678	0.81	0.993	0.993	0.162	0.989	0.91	0	0.984	0.989	0.618	0.973	0.147
12222	0.058	0.037	0.954	0.976	0.015	0.923	0.077	0.016	0	0.921	0.032	0.19	0.006
12211	0.016	0.011	0.942	0.775	0.007	0.364	0.042	0.011	0.079	0	0	0.058	0.005
33212	0.874	0.713	0.991	0.997	0.129	0.995	0.766	0.382	0.968	1	0	0.952	0.028
21312	0.095	0.063	0.979	0.981	0.03	0.902	0.234	0.027	0.81	0.942	0.048	0	0.01
33323	0.973	0.967	0.985	0.997	0.309	0.986	0.931	0.853	0.994	0.995	0.972	0.99	0
33232	0.956	0.928	0.987	0.997	0.247	0.99	0.947	0.765	0.99	0.995	0.912	0.978	0.259
11113	0.181	0.148	0.873	0.967	0.049	0.731	0.196	0.11	0.602	0.765	0.148	0.426	0.033
22323	0.537	0.594	0.99	0.997	0.118	0.99	0.717	0.272	0.964	0.99	0.336	0.937	0.047
32223	0.881	0.817	0.99	0.993	0.183	0.994	0.852	0.597	0.985	0.995	0.664	0.953	0.067
32331	0.968	0.937	0.993	0.993	0.21	0.995	0.964	0.612	0.973	0.989	0.791	0.968	0.207
12223	0.308	0.292	0.979	0.981	0.056	0.958	0.397	0.087	0.949	0.988	0.218	0.707	0.016
11131	0.312	0.291	0.964	0.957	0.073	0.905	0.122	0.048	0.744	0.893	0.253	0.552	0.07
32232	0.919	0.864	1	0.997	0.194	1	0.906	0.479	0.988	0.988	0.644	0.961	0.155
11133	0.482	0.478	0.994	0.977	0.1	0.967	0.627	0.231	0.919	0.968	0.407	0.812	0.131
33321	0.944	0.928	0.993	0.987	0.184	0.984	0.867	0.683	0.972	0.982	0.83	0.97	0.098
22331	0.568	0.667	0.989	0.982	0.13	0.989	0.817	0.201	0.969	0.995	0.418	0.961	0.077
13311	0.36	0.173	0.979	0.983	0.045	0.969	0.415	0.063	0.898	0.968	0.145	0.796	0.027
21323	0.459	0.486	0.986	0.977	0.086	0.982	0.678	0.184	0.969	0.989	0.298	0.882	0.056
12111	0.017	0.007	0.659	0.637	0.003	0.086	0.024	0.007	0.031	0.076	0.003	0.037	0.003
13212	0.232	0.123	0.977	0.99	0.05	0.915	0.286	0.084	0.856	0.966	0.056	0.532	0.02
22233	0.597	0.743	0.994	0.994	0.146	0.99	0.887	0.352	0.984	0.989	0.532	0.909	0.145
32313	0.896	0.876	0.99	0.997	0.157	0.995	0.85	0.663	0.983	0.989	0.735	0.982	0.061

Table 17.5 Scale values computed from implied TTO preferences

State	Thurstone scale value	Transformed Thurstone scale value	Mean observed TTO score	Difference
21111	1.823	0.878	0.878	0.000
11121	1.693	0.830	0.850	0.020
11211	1.677	0.824	0.869	0.045
12111	1.600	0.795	0.834	0.039
11112	1.534	0.771	0.829	0.058
12211	1.315	0.697	0.767	0.070
12121	1.241	0.662	0.742	0.080
11122	1.072	0.599	0.722	0.123
22112	0.949	0.553	0.665	0.112
22121	0.863	0.522	0.642	0.120
21222	0.706	0.463	0.553	0.090
22122	0.667	0.449	0.540	0.091
12222	0.618	0.431	0.551	0.120
21312	0.617	0.430	0.536	0.106
11312	0.612	0.428	0.552	0.124
22222	0.478	0.379	0.500	0.121
13212	0.286	0.307	0.389	0.082
11113	0.278	0.304	0.392	0.088
13311	0.189	0.271	0.346	0.075
12223	-0.098	0.165	0.216	0.051
32211	-0.115	0.158	0.152	-0.006
11131	-0.116	0.158	0.200	0.042
23321	-0.244	0.110	0.147	0.037
21323	-0.279	0.097	0. 160	0.063
21232	-0.404	0.051	0.064	0.013
22323	-0.523	0.007	0.042	0.035
dead	-0.541	0.000	0.000	0.000
33212	-0.586	-0.017	-0.022	-0.005
22331	-0.587	-0.017	-0.011	0.006
11133	-0.595	-0.020	-0.049	-0.029
23313	-0.638	-0.036	-0.070	-0.034
21133	-0.679	-0.051	-0.063	-0.012
23232	-0.716	-0.065	-0.084	-0.019
33321	-0.768	-0.084	-0.120	-0.036
32313	-0.865	-0.120	-0.152	-0.032
22233	-0.903	-0.134	-0.142	-0.008
32223	-0.907	-0.136	-0.174	-0.038
32232	-0.945	-0.150	-0.223	-0.073
13332	-0.991	-0.167	-0.228	-0.061
32331	-1.055	-0.191	-0.276	-0.085
uncon	-1.246	-0.262	-0.402	-0.140
33232	-1.284	-0.276	-0.332	-0.056
33323	-1.308	-0.285	-0.386	-0.101
33333	-1.744	-0.447	-0.543	-0.096

Table 17.6 Computed scale values from ranking task

State	Thurstone scale value	Transformed Thurstone scale value	Mean observed TTO score	Difference
11112	1.9626	0.848	0.829	-0.019
11121	1.9614	0.848	0.850	0.002
11211	1.882	0.829	0.869	0.040
12111	1.8426	0.819	0.834	0.015
21111	1.7655	0.800	0.878	0.078
12211	1.4856	0.733	0.767	0.034
11122	1.4724	0.729	0.722	-0.007
12121	1.4132	0.715	0.742	0.027
22121	1.0613	0.630	0.645	0.015
22112	1.0168	0.619	0.662	0.043
12222	0.9087	0.593	0.551	-0.042
21222	0.7835	0.563	0.553	-0.010
11312	0.7683	0.559	0.552	-0.007
22122	0.7504	0.555	0.540	-0.015
11113	0.5654	0.510	0.392	-0.118
22222	0.5356	0.503	0.500	-0.003
21312	0.4689	0.487	0.536	0.049
13212	0.3096	0.448	0.389	-0.059
11131	0.2918	0.444	0.200	-0.244
12223	0.0909	0.395	0.216	-0.179
13311	0.0142	0.377	0.346	-0.031
21232	-0.1347	0.341	0.064	-0.277
32211	-0.2979	0.301	0.152	-0.149
21323	-0.3307	0.293	0.160	-0.133
11133	-0.3663	0.285	-0.049	-0.334
23321	-0.3847	0.280	0.147	-0.133
21133	-0.5424	0.242	-0.063	-0.305
22331	-0.5784	0.233	-0.01 1	-0.244
22323	-0.6044	0.227	0.042	-0.185
33212	-0.6731	0.211	-0.022	-0.233
23232	-0.6999	0.204	-0.084	-0.288
23313	-0.7869	0.183	-0.070	-0.253
22233	-0.878	0.161	-0.142	-0.303
32232	-0.9158	0.152	-0.174	-0.326
13332	-0.9643	0.140	-0.228	-0.368
32223	-0.9938	0.133	-0.174	-0.307
33321	-1.0579	0.117	-0.120	-0.237
32313	-1.1827	0.087	-0.152	-0.239
32331	-1 .2261	0.077	-0.276	-0.353
33232	-1.3804	0.039	-0.332	-0.371
uncon	-1.5327	0.003	-0.402	-0.405
death	-1 .5437	0.000	0.000	0.000
33323	-1.6146	-0.017	-0.386	-0.369
33333	-2.4053	-0.208	-0.543	-0.335

The close correspondence between mean observed TTO values and those resulting from the two Thurstone models can also be seen in Figure 17.2 and Figure 17.3.

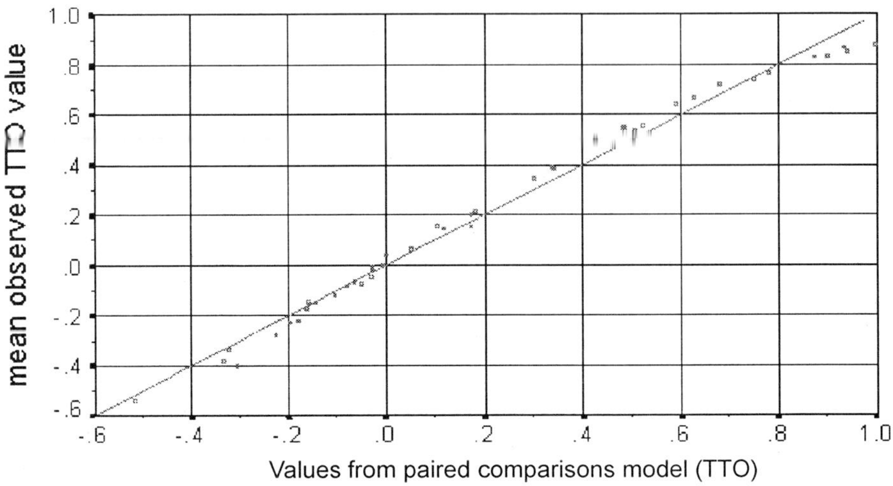

Figure 17.2 Analysis of preferences in TTO data

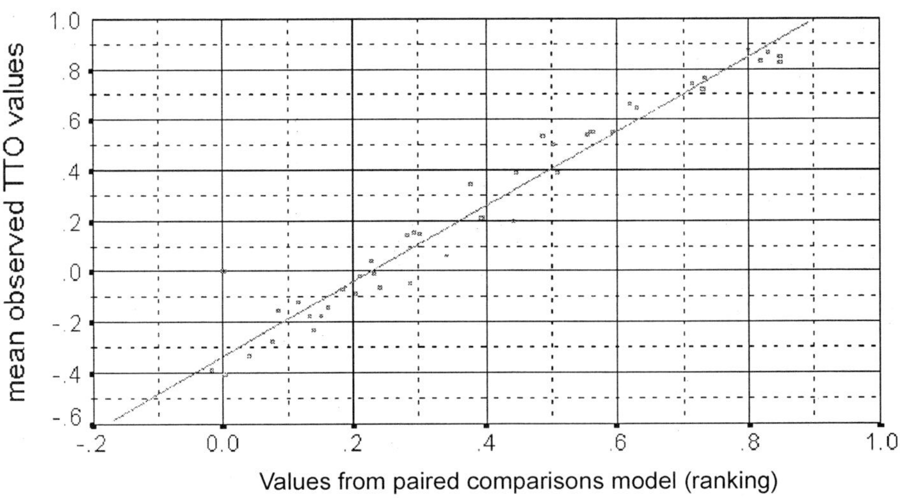

Figure 17.3 Analysis of preferences in ranking data

17.3 INTERPOLATING TARIFF VALUES

Having thus established a functional relationship between the observed and estimated TTO values, further analysis was restricted to the estimated values based on the Thurstone model results. These scores were analysed using the 'N3-model ' (reported in the Second MVH Report, February 1995). This model includes a set of dummy variables for each dimension, indicating movement away from level I (no problem). A further dummy variable indicates the presence of at least 1 dimension with a level 3 descriptor. Table 17.7 gives the decrements which resulted from that regression model to the scale values produced by the paired comparisons models. For completeness these are tablulated with the corresponding decrements associated with the TTO Al tariff. Whilst the decrements for level 2 mobility, pain/discomfort and anxiety/ depression are virtually identical in both models, the relative positions of self-care and usual activity are reversed. Much greater prominence is given to usual activity in the Thurstone-based model. The pattern persists into level 3.

There are systematic differences between the two sets of estimated scale values with results from the ranking task receiving higher values for the more severe states than those which result from the TTO procedure (Figure17.4).

Table 17.7 Decrements for pairwise model tariff and TTO Al tariff

EuroQol dimension	TTO Al tariff		'TTO' tariff estimated from implied preferenes		'TTO' tariff estimated from ranking task	
	level 2	level 3	level 2	level 3	level 2	level 3
Mobility	0.069	0.314	0.066	0.271	0.078	0.228
Self-care	0.104	0.214	0.029	0.097	0.082	0.167
Usual activity	0.036	0.094	0.127	0.224	0.032	0.106
Pain/discomfort	0.121	0.386	0.144	0.376	0.066	0.199
Anxiety/depression	0.074	0.236	0.114	0.259	0.051	0.159
	constant = 0.081 N3 = 0.269		constant = 0.030 N3 = 0.305		constant = 0. 146 N3 0.16	

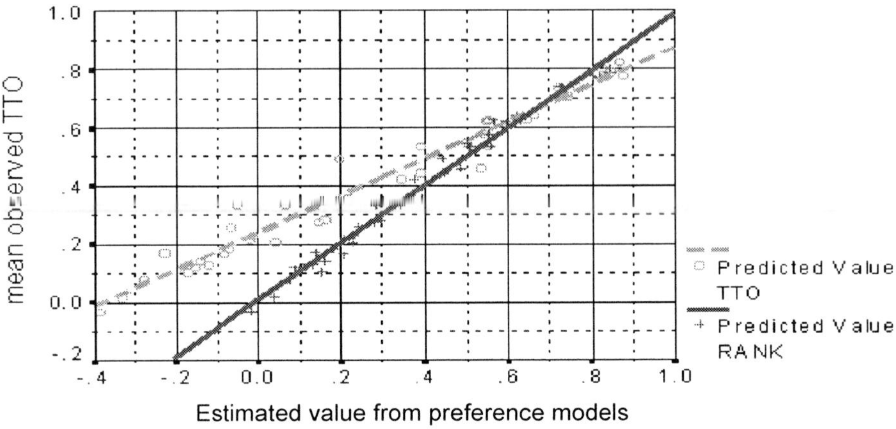

Figure 17.4 Estimated values for directly observed health states based on TTO and ranking preferences

The full tariff of values based on the Thurstone estimates for these models is given in Table 17.8 and 17.9.

Finally, Figure 17.5 brings together the tariff based on the original TTO data generated by the MVH survey, and used in the construction of the Al tariff, with corresponding values estimated from the decrements listed in Table 17.7, and based upon the preference information extracted from the ranking task.

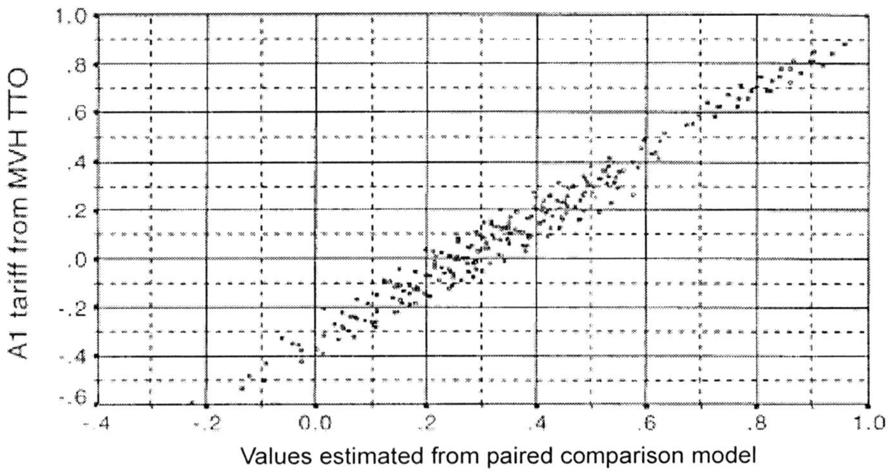

Figure 17.5 Tariff values estimated from the observed TTO data and corresponding values in a tariff estimated from the ranking task

Table 17.8 Tariff of values based on TTO preference matrix

EuroQol dimension	level 2	level 3
Mobility	0.066	0.271
Self-care	0.029	0.097
Usual activities	0.127	0.224
Pain / discomfort	0.144	0.376
Anxiety / depression	0.114	0.259
	constant = 0.030	n3 = 0.305

1 1 1 1 1	1.00	1 2 3 2 2	0.15	2 1 2 3 3	-0.16	2 3 2 2 1	0.23	3 2 1 3 2	-0.12
1 1 1 1 2	0.86	1 2 3 2 3	0.01	2 1 3 1 1	0.38	2 3 2 2 2	0.12	3 2 1 3 3	-0.27
1 1 1 1 3	0.41	1 2 3 3 1	0.04	2 1 3 1 2	0.26	2 3 2 2 3	-0.03	3 2 2 1 1	0.24
1 1 1 2 1	0.83	1 2 3 3 2	-0.08	2 1 3 1 3	0.12	2 3 2 3 1	0.00	3 2 2 1 2	0.12
1 1 1 2 2	0.71	1 2 3 3 3	-0.22	2 1 3 2 1	0.23	2 3 2 3 2	-0.11	3 2 2 1 3	-0.02
1 1 1 2 3	0.26	1 3 1 1 1	0.57	2 1 3 2 2	0.12	2 3 2 3 3	-0.26	3 2 2 2 1	0.09
1 1 1 3 1	0.29	1 3 1 1 2	0.45	2 1 3 2 3	-0.03	2 3 3 1 1	0.28	3 2 2 2 2	-0.02
1 1 1 3 2	0.18	1 3 1 1 3	0.31	2 1 3 3 1	0.00	2 3 3 1 2	0.16	3 2 2 2 3	-0.17
1 1 1 3 3	0.03	1 3 1 2 1	0.42	2 1 3 3 2	-0.11	2 3 3 1 3	0.02	3 2 2 3 1	-0.14
1 1 2 1 1	0.84	1 3 1 2 2	0.31	2 1 3 3 3	-0.26	2 3 3 2 1	0.13	3 2 2 3 2	-0.25
1 1 2 1 2	0.73	1 3 1 2 3	0.17	2 2 1 1 1	0.88	2 3 3 2 2	0.02	3 2 2 3 3	-0.40
1 1 2 1 3	0.28	1 3 1 3 1	0.19	2 2 1 1 2	0.76	2 3 3 2 3	-0.12	3 2 3 1 1	0.14
1 1 2 2 1	0.70	1 3 1 3 2	0.08	2 2 1 1 3	0.31	2 3 3 3 1	-0.10	3 2 3 1 2	0.03
1 1 2 2 2	0.59	1 3 1 3 3	-0.07	2 2 1 2 1	0.73	2 3 3 3 2	-0.21	3 2 3 1 3	-0.12
1 1 2 2 3	0.14	1 3 2 1 1	0.44	2 2 1 2 2	0.62	2 3 3 3 3	-0.36	3 2 3 2 1	0.00
1 1 2 3 1	0.16	1 3 2 1 2	0.33	2 2 1 2 3	0.17	3 1 1 1 1	0.39	3 2 3 2 2	-0.12
1 1 2 3 2	0.05	1 3 2 1 3	0.18	2 2 1 3 1	0.19	3 1 1 1 2	0.28	3 2 3 2 3	-0.26
1 1 2 3 3	-0.10	1 3 2 2 1	0.30	2 2 1 3 2	0.08	3 1 1 1 3	0.13	3 2 3 3 1	-0.23
1 1 3 1 1	0.44	1 3 2 2 2	0.18	2 2 1 3 3	-0.06	3 1 1 2 1	0.25	3 2 3 3 2	-0.35
1 1 3 1 2	0.33	1 3 2 2 3	0.04	2 2 2 1 1	0.75	3 1 1 2 2	0.14	3 2 3 3 3	-0.49
1 1 3 1 3	0.18	1 3 2 3 1	0.07	2 2 2 1 2	0.63	3 1 1 2 3	-0.01	3 3 1 1 1	0.30
1 1 3 2 1	0.30	1 3 2 3 2	-0.05	2 2 2 1 3	0.18	3 1 1 3 1	0.02	3 3 1 1 2	0.18
1 1 3 2 2	0.18	1 3 2 3 3	-0.19	2 2 2 2 1	0.60	3 1 1 3 2	-0.10	3 3 1 1 3	0.04
1 1 3 2 3	0.04	1 3 3 1 1	0.34	2 2 2 2 2	0.49	3 1 1 3 3	-0.24	3 3 1 2 1	0.15
1 1 3 3 1	0.07	1 3 3 1 2	0.23	2 2 2 2 3	0.04	3 1 2 1 1	0.27	3 3 1 2 2	0.04
1 1 3 3 2	-0.05	1 3 3 1 3	0.09	2 2 2 3 1	0.07	3 1 2 1 2	0.15	3 3 1 2 3	-0.11
1 1 3 3 3	-0.19	1 3 3 2 1	0.20	2 2 2 3 2	-0.05	3 1 2 1 3	0.01	3 3 1 3 1	-0.08
1 2 1 1 1	0.94	1 3 3 2 2	0.09	2 2 2 3 3	-0.19	3 1 2 2 1	0.12	3 3 1 3 2	-0.19
1 2 1 1 2	0.83	1 3 3 2 3	-0.06	2 2 3 1 1	0.35	3 1 2 2 2	0.01	3 3 1 3 3	-0.34
1 2 1 1 3	0.38	1 3 3 3 1	-0.03	2 2 3 1 2	0.23	3 1 2 2 3	-0.14	3 3 2 1 1	0.17
1 2 1 2 1	0.80	1 3 3 3 2	-0.15	2 2 3 1 3	0.09	3 1 2 3 1	-0.11	3 3 2 1 2	0.06
1 2 1 2 2	0.68	1 3 3 3 3	-0.29	2 2 3 2 1	0.20	3 1 2 3 2	-0.22	3 3 2 1 3	-0.09
1 2 1 2 3	0.23	2 1 1 1 1	0.90	2 2 3 2 2	0.09	3 1 2 3 3	-0.37	3 3 2 2 1	0.03
1 2 1 3 1	0.26	2 1 1 1 2	0.79	2 2 3 2 3	-0.06	3 1 3 1 1	0.17	3 3 2 2 2	-0.09
1 2 1 3 2	0.15	2 1 1 1 3	0.34	2 2 3 3 1	-0.03	3 1 3 1 2	0.06	3 3 2 2 3	-0.23
1 2 1 3 3	0.00	2 1 1 2 1	0.76	2 2 3 3 2	-0.14	3 1 3 1 3	-0.09	3 3 2 3 1	-0.21
1 2 2 1 1	0.81	2 1 1 2 2	0.65	2 2 3 3 3	-0.29	3 1 3 2 1	0.03	3 3 2 3 2	-0.32
1 2 2 1 2	0.70	2 1 1 2 3	0.20	2 3 1 1 1	0.50	3 1 3 2 2	-0.09	3 3 2 3 3	-0.47
1 2 2 1 3	0.25	2 1 1 3 1	0.22	2 3 1 1 2	0.39	3 1 3 2 3	-0.23	3 3 3 1 1	0.07
1 2 2 2 1	0.67	2 1 1 3 2	0.11	2 3 1 1 3	0.24	3 1 3 3 1	-0.21	3 3 3 1 2	-0.04
1 2 2 2 2	0.56	2 1 1 3 3	-0.04	2 3 1 2 1	0.36	3 1 3 3 2	-0.32	3 3 3 1 3	-0.19
1 2 2 2 3	0.11	2 1 2 1 1	0.78	2 3 1 2 2	0.24	3 1 3 3 3	-0.47	3 3 3 2 1	-0.07
1 2 2 3 1	0.13	2 1 2 1 2	0.66	2 3 1 2 3	0.10	3 2 1 1 1	0.37	3 3 3 2 2	-0.19
1 2 2 3 2	0.02	2 1 2 1 3	0.21	2 3 1 3 1	0.13	3 2 1 1 2	0.25	3 3 3 2 3	-0.33
1 2 2 3 3	-0.13	2 1 2 2 1	0.63	2 3 1 3 2	0.01	3 2 1 1 3	0.11	3 3 3 3 1	-0.30
1 2 3 1 1	0.41	2 1 2 2 2	0.52	2 3 1 3 3	-0.13	3 2 1 2 1	0.22	3 3 3 3 2	-0.42
1 2 3 1 2	0.30	2 1 2 2 3	0.07	2 3 2 1 1	0.38	3 2 1 2 2	0.11	3 3 3 3 3	-0.56
1 2 3 1 3	0.15	2 1 2 3 1	0.10	2 3 2 1 2	0.26	3 2 1 2 3	-0.04	unconscious	-0.28
1 2 3 2 1	0.27	2 1 2 3 2	-0.02	2 3 2 1 3	0.12	3 2 1 3 1	-0.01		

Table 17.9 Tariff of values derived from ranking preferences

EuroQol dimension	level 2	level 3
Mobility	0.078	0.228
Self-care	0.032	0.106
Usual activities	0.082	0.167
Pain / discomfort	0.066	0.199
Anxiety / depression	0.051	0.159
	constant = 0.146	n3 = 0.161

1 1 1 1 1	1.000	1 2 3 2 2	0.377	2 1 2 3 3	0.175	2 3 2 2 1	0.361	3 2 1 3 2	0.183
1 1 1 1 2	0.803	1 2 3 2 3	0.269	2 1 3 1 1	0.448	2 3 2 2 2	0.310	3 2 1 3 3	0.075
1 1 1 1 3	0.534	1 2 3 3 1	0.295	2 1 3 1 2	0.397	2 3 2 2 3	0.202	3 2 2 1 1	0.351
1 1 1 2 1	0.788	1 2 3 3 2	0.244	2 1 3 1 3	0.289	2 3 2 3 1	0.228	3 2 2 1 2	0.300
1 1 1 2 2	0.737	1 2 3 3 3	0.136	2 1 3 2 1	0.382	2 3 2 3 2	0.177	3 2 2 1 3	0.192
1 1 1 2 3	0.468	1 3 1 1 1	0.587	2 1 3 2 2	0.331	2 3 2 3 3	0.069	3 2 2 2 1	0.285
1 1 1 3 1	0.494	1 3 1 1 2	0.536	2 1 3 2 3	0.223	2 3 3 1 1	0.342	3 2 2 2 2	0.234
1 1 1 3 2	0.443	1 3 1 1 3	0.428	2 1 3 3 1	0.249	2 3 3 1 2	0.291	3 2 2 2 3	0.126
1 1 1 3 3	0.335	1 3 1 2 1	0.521	2 1 3 3 2	0.198	2 3 3 1 3	0.183	3 2 2 3 1	0.152
1 1 2 1 1	0.772	1 3 1 2 2	0.470	2 1 3 3 3	0.090	2 3 3 2 1	0.276	3 2 2 3 2	0.101
1 1 2 1 2	0.721	1 3 1 2 3	0.362	2 2 1 1 1	0.744	2 3 3 2 2	0.225	3 2 2 3 3	-0.007
1 1 2 1 3	0.452	1 3 1 3 1	0.388	2 2 1 1 2	0.693	2 3 3 2 3	0.117	3 2 3 1 1	0.266
1 1 2 2 1	0.706	1 3 1 3 2	0.337	2 2 1 1 3	0.424	2 3 3 3 1	0.143	3 2 3 1 2	0.215
1 1 2 2 2	0.655	1 3 1 3 3	0.229	2 2 1 2 1	0.678	2 3 3 3 2	0.092	3 2 3 1 3	0.107
1 1 2 2 3	0.386	1 3 2 1 1	0.505	2 2 1 2 2	0.627	2 3 3 3 3	-0.016	3 2 3 2 1	0.200
1 1 2 3 1	0.412	1 3 2 1 2	0.454	2 2 1 2 3	0.358	3 1 1 1 1	0.465	3 2 3 2 2	0.149
1 1 2 3 2	0.361	1 3 2 1 3	0.346	2 2 1 3 1	0.384	3 1 1 1 2	0.414	3 2 3 2 3	0.041
1 1 2 3 3	0.253	1 3 2 2 1	0.439	2 2 1 3 2	0.333	3 1 1 1 3	0.306	3 2 3 3 1	0.067
1 1 3 1 1	0.526	1 3 2 2 2	0.388	2 2 1 3 3	0.225	3 1 1 2 1	0.399	3 2 3 3 2	0.016
1 1 3 1 2	0.475	1 3 2 2 3	0.280	2 2 2 1 1	0.662	3 1 1 2 2	0.348	3 2 3 3 3	-0.092
1 1 3 1 3	0.367	1 3 2 3 1	0.306	2 2 2 1 2	0.611	3 1 1 2 3	0.240	3 3 1 1 1	0.359
1 1 3 2 1	0.460	1 3 2 3 2	0.255	2 2 2 1 3	0.342	3 1 1 3 1	0.266	3 3 1 1 2	0.308
1 1 3 2 2	0.409	1 3 2 3 3	0.147	2 2 2 2 1	0.596	3 1 1 3 2	0.215	3 3 1 1 3	0.200
1 1 3 2 3	0.301	1 3 3 1 1	0.420	2 2 2 2 2	0.545	3 1 1 3 3	0.107	3 3 1 2 1	0.293
1 1 3 3 1	0.327	1 3 3 1 2	0.369	2 2 2 2 3	0.276	3 1 2 1 1	0.383	3 3 1 2 2	0.242
1 1 3 3 2	0.276	1 3 3 1 3	0.261	2 2 2 3 1	0.302	3 1 2 1 2	0.332	3 3 1 2 3	0.134
1 1 3 3 3	0.168	1 3 3 2 1	0.354	2 2 2 3 2	0.251	3 1 2 1 3	0.224	3 3 1 3 1	0.160
1 2 1 1 1	0.822	1 3 3 2 2	0.303	2 2 2 3 3	0.143	3 1 2 2 1	0.317	3 3 1 3 2	0.109
1 2 1 1 2	0.771	1 3 3 2 3	0.195	2 2 3 1 1	0.416	3 1 2 2 2	0.266	3 3 1 3 3	0.001
1 2 1 1 3	0.502	1 3 3 3 1	0.221	2 2 3 1 2	0.365	3 1 2 2 3	0.158	3 3 2 1 1	0.277
1 2 1 2 1	0.756	1 3 3 3 2	0.170	2 2 3 1 3	0.257	3 1 2 3 1	0.184	3 3 2 1 2	0.226
1 2 1 2 2	0.705	1 3 3 3 3	0.062	2 2 3 2 1	0.350	3 1 2 3 2	0.133	3 3 2 1 3	0.118
1 2 1 2 3	0.436	2 1 1 1 1	0.776	2 2 3 2 2	0.299	3 1 2 3 3	0.025	3 3 2 2 1	0.211
1 2 1 3 1	0.462	2 1 1 1 2	0.725	2 2 3 2 3	0.191	3 1 3 1 1	0.298	3 3 2 2 2	0.160
1 2 1 3 2	0.411	2 1 1 1 3	0.456	2 2 3 3 1	0.217	3 1 3 1 2	0.247	3 3 2 2 3	0.052
1 2 1 3 3	0.303	2 1 1 2 1	0.710	2 2 3 3 2	0.166	3 1 3 1 3	0.139	3 3 2 3 1	0.078
1 2 2 1 1	0.740	2 1 1 2 2	0.659	2 2 3 3 3	0.058	3 1 3 2 1	0.232	3 3 2 3 2	0.027
1 2 2 1 2	0.689	2 1 1 2 3	0.390	2 3 1 1 1	0.509	3 1 3 2 2	0.181	3 3 2 3 3	-0.081
1 2 2 1 3	0.420	2 1 1 3 1	0.416	2 3 1 1 2	0.458	3 1 3 2 3	0.073	3 3 3 1 1	0.192
1 2 2 2 1	0.674	2 1 1 3 2	0.365	2 3 1 1 3	0.350	3 1 3 3 1	0.099	3 3 3 1 2	0.141
1 2 2 2 2	0.623	2 1 1 3 3	0.257	2 3 1 2 1	0.443	3 1 3 3 2	0.048	3 3 3 1 3	0.033
1 2 2 2 3	0.354	2 1 2 1 1	0.694	2 3 1 2 2	0.392	3 1 3 3 3	-0.060	3 3 3 2 1	0.126
1 2 2 3 1	0.380	2 1 2 1 2	0.643	2 3 1 2 3	0.284	3 2 1 1 1	0.433	3 3 3 2 2	0.075
1 2 2 3 2	0.329	2 1 2 1 3	0.374	2 3 1 3 1	0.310	3 2 1 1 2	0.382	3 3 3 2 3	-0.033
1 2 2 3 3	0.221	2 1 2 2 1	0.628	2 3 1 3 2	0.259	3 2 1 1 3	0.274	3 3 3 3 1	-0.007
1 2 3 1 1	0.494	2 1 2 2 2	0.577	2 3 1 3 3	0.151	3 2 1 2 1	0.367	3 3 3 3 2	-0.058
1 2 3 1 2	0.443	2 1 2 2 3	0.308	2 3 2 1 1	0.427	3 2 1 2 2	0.316	3 3 3 3 3	-0.166
1 2 3 1 3	0.335	2 1 2 3 1	0.334	2 3 2 1 2	0.376	3 2 1 2 3	0.208		
1 2 3 2 1	0.428	2 1 2 3 2	0.283	2 3 2 1 3	0.268	3 2 1 3 1	0.234		

17.4 SUMMARY

Working on the assumption that the data produced by TTO yields only ordinal information rather than cardinal information, we have processed the data according to a well-established model that is known to yield an interval scale. These modelled scale values can be reliably converted into values that correspond to a remarkable degree with the mean TTO values. Utilising these values recovered from the preference information contained within the TTO data leads to a tariff of values which broadly approximates to the original Al tariff. Similar results have been previously obtained using ordinal information recovered from quantitative data - see for example, the results of analysing magnitude estimation values as categorical data (Kind, 1981).

Given the proximity of the estimated values to those actually observed in the TTO data, it seems as though this is no chance phenomenon. If that is so, then we must seek an explanation for the Thurstone model's capacity to recover cardinal information from ordinal preferences. Thurstone Case V relies upon the similarity in standard deviation of the discriminal process for all states. This may be something of an heroic assumption, and estimates of their magnitude are needed before accepting the results of the analysis presented above. Indications suggest that this assumption holds for most states until moderate to extreme severity is encountered. The model is based upon the notion of a single dimensioned valuation continuum and if the evidence of this analysis is confirmed, then it may be safely taken that health state valuations may be represented by a single index score (even those based upon composite health state descriptions). Furthermore, this result tends to support the assertion that TTO values lie on a true cardinal scale, with interval scale properties.

Paired comparisons methods require either a large number of judgements from individual subjects, or single observations from a large number of subjects. In general, n states generates $n \cdot (n - 1) / 2$ comparisons and Torgerson (1958) describes several experimental techniques for avoiding an excessive burden on researchers or subjects in their studies. These include ranking and sorting techniques which yield similar results to those obtained from conventional paired comparisons

Paired comparisons models (of which the original Thurstone variant is but one) sometimes suffer from their inability to cope with extreme preferences. Where health states tend to be always regarded as more severe than other states, for example the state 33333, then some form of data censoring may be needed to enable the computational process to proceed. A variety of strategies exist for coping with missing elements in the P-matrix which result from such exclusions. Alternative models have been proposed in which other forms of distributions substitute for the unit normal distribution used in the Thurstone model.

The measurement of health state valuations often necessitates complex tasks that stretch an individual's intellectual processes - and sometimes appear to offer challenges that defy all but the most able and imaginative of judges. Perhaps it is time to reconsider the possibilities offered by a far simpler procedure.

Original report prepared for the EuroQol Plenary Meeting: Oslo, Norway, 1996

17.5 REFERENCES

Edwards. Techniques of attitude scale construction. New Jersey: Prentice-Hall, 1957.

Fanshel S, Bush J W. A health status index and its application to health services outcomes. Operations Research 1970;18:1021.

Kind P. A comparison of two models for scaling health indicators. International Journal of Epidemiology 1982;11(3):271-275.

Kind P, Rosser R M. The quantification of health. European Journal of Social Psychology 1988;18(1):63-77.

MeKenna S, Hunt S M, McEwen J. Weighting the seriousness of perceived health problems using Thurstone's method of paired comparisons. International Journal of Epidemiology 1981;10:93-97.

Thurstone L L. A law of comparative judgement. Psychological Review 1927;34:273-286.

Thurstone L L. Attitudes can be measured. American Journal of Sociology 1928;33:529-554.

Torgerson W S. Theory and methods of scaling. New York: John Wiley, 1958.

18
The use and usefulness of the EuroQol EQ-5D: preliminary results from an international survey

Rosalind Rabin, Paul Kind and Frank de Charro

18.1 BACKGROUND

Since the introduction of the EuroQol Instrument into the public domain in 1990, the EQ-5D and its predecessor, the EQ-6D, has been used by an increasing number of researchers, clinicians and the pharmaceutical industry. Some, but by no means all, of these applications involve members of the EuroQol Group, either working directly in collaboration, or in an advisory role.

The EuroQol Foundation was formally established in 1995. Its functions include providing an organisation responsible for the effective dissemination of up to date information concerning the EQ-5D. This is clearly important for those researchers and clinicians who are currently using the EQ-5D but would like to learn more about its use by others in the same field of inquiry. It is also recognised that many researchers who are using the EQ-5D would appreciate contact with other groups who are using the instrument in a similar clinical area. The need to acquire accurate information will be of particular interest to those who adopted early versions of the instrument and who are now in the process of analysing their data.

By the beginning of 1996, the Group was aware of studies using the EQ-5D in several European countries as well as in North America. The studies encompassed a wide number of different clinical areas. However, while some studies were well known particularly to the EuroQol Group and especially those carried out by Group members or their institutions, much of the evidence was informal. It was decided that a more systematic investigation of the use and usefulness of the instrument needed to be undertaken.

18.2 THE SURVEY

In May 1996, a brief three page form together with an explanatory covering letter, was distributed to 369 addresses comprising mainly health services researchers, clinicians and the pharmaceutical industry. A copy of the form is attached as Appendix 18.1. The contacts included people on the EuroQol Business Management mailing list who had expressed an interest in the Group's work, together with contacts from the Centre for Health Economics, University of York, UK. The information was requested by 21st June 1996. No follow-up letter or reminder was sent. A further mailing to 50 additional addressees was sent from York in August 1996

P. Kind et al. (eds.), EQ-5D concepts and methods, 221–234.

From a total of 419 people mailed, 120 (29%) responded. 64 people said they were using the EQ-5D in 84 different studies. 3 forms were returned undelivered.

A follow-up of EuroQol Group members, based on Paul Kind's "in-house" survey of May 1996, elicited 29 further studies being undertaken by Group members or their institutions. Telephone or e-mail follow-up with approximately 14 non-EuroQol Group members elicited a further 19 studies. Therefore, 132 studies using the EQ-5D were identified.

Three people indicated that they were not prepared to have their studies included in a report of the survey and one person indicated that he was not prepared to have his contact details published in the survey to facilitate contact with other research colleagues. Two people indicated they were not prepared to permit either publication of their study nor contact details.

Studies have been preliminarily grouped into clinical areas based on medical textbook classifications and Berzon's cumulative index to quality of life instruments by therapeutic category (Berzon *et al*, 1995).

Figure 18.1 shows the clinical areas covered. A more detailed breakdown showing study titles within each clinical area is contained in Appendix 18.2. Numbers of studies involved are shown in Table 18.1.

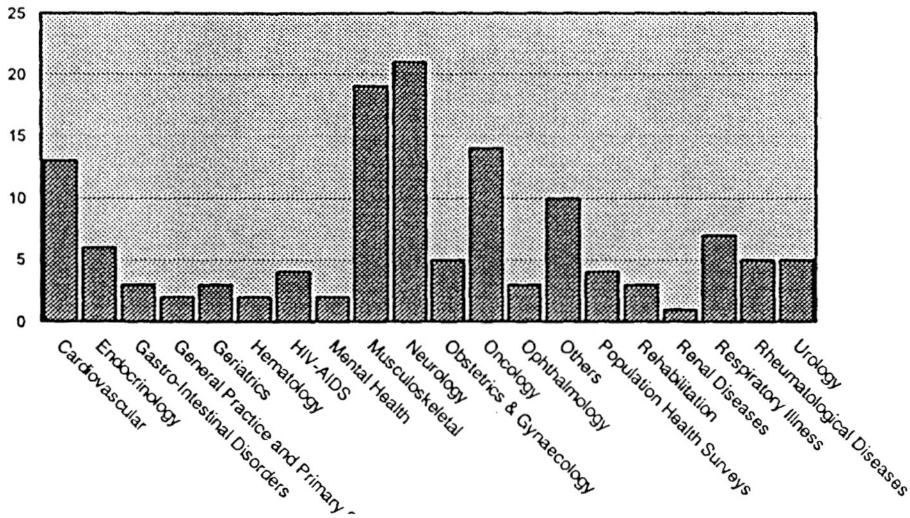

Figure 18.1 Results from an international survey showing 19 clinical areas covered by the EQ-5D

Table 18.1 Number of studies using the EQ-5D defined by clinical area

Clinical Area	Total
Cardiovascular	13
Endocrinology	6
Gastro-intestinal Disorders	3
General Practice & Primary Care	2
Geriatrics	3
Hematology	2
HIV-AIDS	4
Mental health	2
Musculoskeletal	19
Neurology	21
Obstetrics & Gynaecology	5
Oncology	14
Ophthalmology	3
Population Health Surveys	4
Rehabilitation	3
Renal Diseases	1
Respiratory Illness	7
Rheumatological Diseases	5
Urology	5
Others	10
Grand Total	132

Information regarding where the studies using the EQ-5D are being undertaken is shown in Figure 18.2. The numbers involved are shown in Table 18.2.

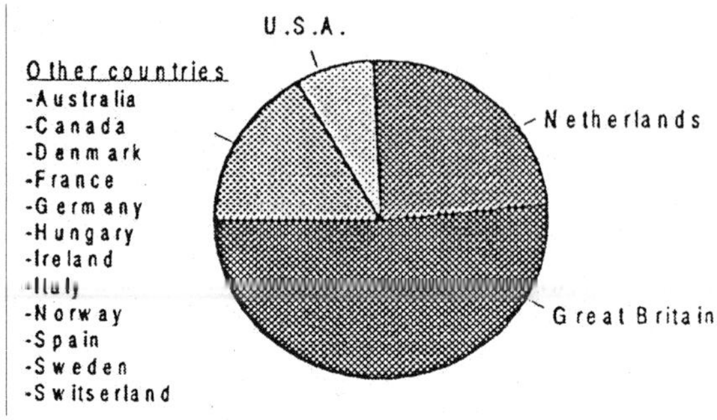

Figure 18.2 Results from an international survey showing areas where studies using the EQ-5D are being undertaken

Table 18.2 Number of studies using the EQ-5D identified within different countries

Countries	Total
Australia	1
Canada	3
Denmark	4
France	2
Germany	2
Great Britain	68
Hungary	1
Ireland	1
Italy	2
Netherlands	32
Norway	1
Spain	1
Sweden	2
Switzerland	2
USA	10
Grand total	132

Details of the type of studies are contained in Figure 18.3. The numbers involved are shown in Table 18.3.

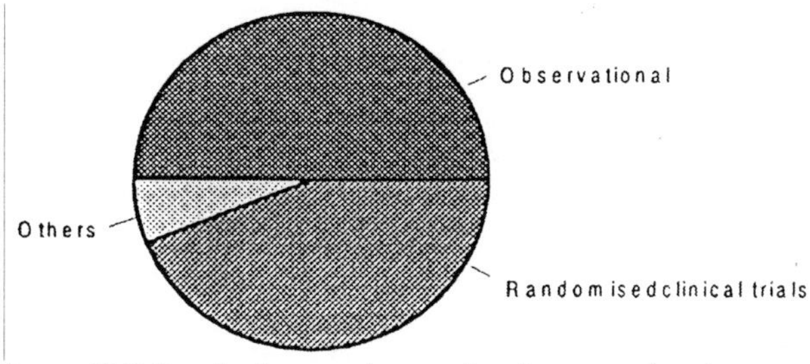

Figure 18.3 Results from an international survey showing types of studies using the EQ-5D

Table 18.3 Number of studies incorporating the EQ-5D defined by study design

Study Design	Total
Observational	66
RCTs	58
Others	8
Grand Total	132

Table 18.4 indicates the sources of funding for studies using the EQ-5D.

Table 18.4 Sources of funding for studies incorporating the EQ-5D

Source of funding	Total
Dutch Health Insurance Board	9
European	4
Government (GB)	24
Government (NL)	8
Government (other than in GB & NL)	2
Medical Research Council (GB)	9
Pharmaceutical industry	18
Regional (GB)	16
Regional (other than in GB)	5
University (GB)	5
University (other than in GB)	6
Others	17
Unknown or unspecified	9
Grand total	132

Table 18.5 shows the generic instruments used alongside the EQ-5D.

Table 18.5 Generic instruments used alongside the EQ-5D (most studies incorporate more than one instrument)

Generic instruments used alongside EQ-5D	Total
Barthel	4
COOP charts	7
FLP	2
HUI	5
Karnofsky	4
NHP	11
QWB	4
SF-36	29
SIP	10

18.3 FUTURE WORK

The report presented here is a preliminary progress report for information of EuroQol Group members only. Since the report has been prepared, more information arising from the survey has been received and will be included in a final report to be circulated at the end of 1996 to EuroQol members and non-members on the mailing list. Other information from the survey data will be analysed and added such as information regarding the use of condition-specific measures being used alongside the EQ-5D, the institutions carrying out the studies, the numbers of patients/people involved as well as information regarding the start and finish dates of the studies. The information reported here has been incorporated into a poster and will be presented at the ISOQOL meeting in Manila, Philippines on the 24-27 October 1996. Efforts will be made by the EuroQol Foundation to regularly update the survey so that accurate information regarding EQ-5D usage can be disseminated in the future.

Original report prepared for the EuroQol Plenary Meeting: Oslo, Norway, 1996

18.4 REFERENCE

Berzon R A, Donnelly M A, Simpson R L, et al. Quality of life bibliography and indexes: 1994 update. Quality of Life Research 1995;4:547-569.

APPENDIX 18.1

THREE PAGE FORM - PAGE 1 OF 3

The EuroQol Foundation

Stadhuisplein 4, 3311 CR Dordrecht, The Netherlands
(Tel:+31 10 4081545/+31 78 6318977) (Fax:+31 78 6350811)
(E-mail:Rabin@GBR.FRG.EUR.NL)

Please can you complete this form and return it in the envelope provided. We have included two additional forms in case you have any research colleagues who may be using or thinking of using the EQ-5D. We would like to receive your replies by 21st June 1996 if possible. If you have any inquiries, please tel/fax/E-mail Rosalind Rabin at the EuroQol Foundation (details above).

For the purposes of updating our records, please could you provide us with the following information:

Name (please print): ______________________________

Affiliation: ______________________________

Postal address: ______________________________

____

____

City: ______________________________

Postal/Zip code: ______________________________

Country: ______________________________

Telephone number(s): ______________________________

Fax number(s): ______________________________

E-mail address: ______________________________

PAGE 2 OF 3

Please complete a separate form for each study involving the EQ-5D

Title of study: ________________________________

____

____

Study objective: ________________________________

____

____

____

____

____

Source(s) of funding: ________________________________

____

____

Study design:
(please give brief details, for example, RCT/observational)

____

____

____

____

____

____

Number of patients: ____________________

PAGE 3/3

Use of other health status measures

Generic	Disease/condition specific

Start/finish dates (planned or actual)

Start: ____________________

Finish: ____________________

Journal articles or other published reports
(please give citation details) (copies would be welcome)

____

____

____

Additional comments

____

____

Are you prepared to have this information included in the report of this survey?

Yes ☐ No ☐

Would you like to have your contact details published in the survey report to facilitate contact with other research colleagues?

Yes ☐ No ☐

Please return this form to: Rosalind Rabin, Management Assistant, the EuroQol Foundation, Stadhuisplein 4, 3311 CR, Dordrecht, The Netherlands.

Thank you for your help

APPENDIX 18.2

TITLES OF ELICITED STUDIES AS DEFINED BY CLINICAL AREA

Cardiovascular

Assessment of two treatment options in the prevention (secondary) of vascular disease
Quality of life, outcome indicators and cost-effectiveness of vascular surgery
Quality of life assessment in patients with peripheral arterial disease
Quality of life in patients treated with pacing
Quality of life in patients with neromediated syncope
Assessment of GP referral of patients with suspected cardiac pathology to a cardiology outpatient clinic
Quality of life after cardiac surgery
The effects of a congestive heart failure clinic on quality of life and functional status
The use of orgal magnesium therapy in mild to moderate congestive heart failure
Validation of the Danish EuroQol questionnaire on patients with acute myocardial infarction
Quality of life after myocardial infarction
Retrospective audit of patients with myocardial infarction seen by coronary heart disease liaison nurse
Secondary heart integrated care project (SHIP)

Endocrinology

Developing outcome measures for ambulatory care - an application to diabetes
Diacom:Evaluation of computer aided nutrition education in diabetes mellitus
Evaluation of treatment of patients with non-insulin dependent diabetes mellitus (NID-FDM) quality of life in short adults
Quality of life in patients with diabetes mellitus type 1
Validation of the Danish EuroQol questionnaire on patients with diabetes

Gastro-intestinal Disorders

A cost-utility analysis of home parenteral nutrition (HPN)
Comparison of health measures in patients with liver disease
Economic evaluation of liver transplantation

General Practice and Primary Care

Comparison of the cost-effectiveness of GPs and nurses for patients requesting a same day appointment
EQ-5D use in a primary care setting

Geriatrics

QUALIDO VIE programme: Quality of life of elderly patients in a rehabilitation unit after hip fracture
QUALIDO VIE programme: Quality of life of the healthy and frail elderly
Using the SF36 and EuroQol on an elderly female population

Hematology

Autologous blood transfusion in total knee replacement surgery
Economic evaluation of alternative transfusion strategies in critical care patients in intensive care units

HIV-AIDS

Assessment of the efficacy of a protease inhibitor in treating HIV infection
Estimating health-related quality of life among persons with HIV infection
Optimising therapy for viral hepatitis in patients with HIV infection
Assessment of treatment in preventing TB in HIV patients

Mental Health

Quality of life of alcohol-dependent patients and their dependants
Validation of the Danish EuroQol questionnaire on patients with depression

Musculoskeletal

Assessment of acupuncture in the treatment of tennis elbow
The spine stabilisation trial
Assessment of the influence of GP referral for X-rays for patients with low back pain
Is the outcome for patients with low back pain influenced by GPs referral for plain radiography?
Primary care management of back pain
Assessment of different treatment options for patients with Colles fracture
The use of growth hormones after hip fracture
Comparison of outcome measures in osteoarthritis
Oefentherapie project. Comparison of treatment options for patients with arthritis
Cost-effectiveness of hip replacement
Quality of life before and after hip replacement in relation to time spent on the waiting list
Joint replacement referral study
Cost-effectiveness of magnetic resonance imaging (MRI) for investigating the knee joint
Cost-effectiveness of magnetic resonance imaging (MRI) for investigating the knee joint
Measuring changes in quality of life following magnetic resonance imaging (MRI) of the knee

Evaluation of referrals by physiotherapists of defined musculoskeletal disorders to orthopaedic clinics
Orthopaedic medicine. Evaluation of a new service
Evaluation of the effect of long term hormone replacement therapy on the development of osteoporosis
Evaluation of laparoscopic surgical repair for inguinal hernia

Neurology

Assessment of magnetic resonance imaging evaluation (MRI) in neurology
Cost-effectiveness of micro-surgery versus radio surgery for acoustic neurinoma
Impact of multiple sclerosis on quality of life
Preliminary assessment of quality of life of people with multiple sclerosis and their carers
Comparison of two treatment options for patients attending neuro-muscular disease clinics
Cost utility analysis of the treatment of dystonia using botulinum toxin
Comparison of discrete choice conjoint and conditional utility modeling using hypertensive veterans
Assessment of outcome measures to examine quality of life in patients with sinus thrombosis
Assessment of two treatment options in the prevention of cerebrovascular disease
Evaluation of domiciliary occupational therapy for stroke patients discharged from hospital
Measuring quality of life in stroke patients
Quality of life assessment in stroke prevention
Quality of life in epilepsy patients awaiting surgery
Audit of anti-epileptic drugs
Cochlear implantation for marginal hearing aid users
Quality of life of patients with dementia
Evaluation of a new treatment on the course of dementia
Quality of life of patients with Gilles de Ia Tourette
Should GPs manage chronic fatigue syndrome?
The impact of migraine on health status
Effectiveness of first-aid as given by a hele-trauma team

Obstetrics & Gynaecology

An economic evaluation of two treatment options in the treatment of menorrhagia
Evaluation of the provision of information and eliciting treatment preferences from women with menorrhagia
Evaluation of a hysterectomy trial
Cost-effectiveness of strategies to prevent neural tube defects
Measuring the effects of a new gynaecological product on older women

Oncology

Quality of life and economic assessment of high dose chemotherapy for oncology patients
Assessment of treatment option for patients with chemotherapy-related febrile neutropenia
Adjuvent breast cancer trial
Start trial - standardisation of breast radiotherapy
Assessment of the impact of breast screening on quality of life valuations
Economic evaluation of chemotherapy for breast cancer
Economic evaluation of intensive chemotherapy for high risk breast cancer
Evaluation of guidelines for the referral and management of breast disorders
Cost-effectiveness of a treatment option for elderly patients with acute myeloid leukaemia
Cost-effectiveness of two treatment options for patients with malignant non-Hodgkin's lymphoma
Evaluation of screening for prostate cancer in age group 55-70 years
Quality of life effects of screening patients with prostate cancer
Technology assessment in colorectal cancer
Utility measurement in patients with lung cancer

Ophthalmology

General health status in relation to visual impairment
Study of Grave's eye disease
The benefits of second eye cataract surgery

Population Health Surveys

Health survey for England 1996
Health status of the British adult population: Omnibus sample survey 1995
Health status of the British adult population: Omnibus sample survey 1996
Somerset and Avon survey of health

Rehabilitation

Analysis of rehabilitation
Cost-effective rehabilitation technology through appropriate indicators (TIDE programme) (Sweden)
Cost-effective rehabilitation technology through appropriate indicators (TIDE programme) (Italy)

Renal Disease

Measuring utilities in an end-stage renal disease population

Respiratory Illness

Quality of life of patients with chronic sinusitis
A pilot study of caring for ventilated patients in the community
Comparison of outcome measures in chronic obstructive pulmonary disease (COPD)
Developing outcome measures for ambulatory care - an application to asthma
Cost effectiveness study of treatment for lung embolism
Economic evaluation of lung transplantation
Assessment of lung transplantation for patients with cystic fibrosis

Rheumatological Diseases

Assessment of the use of utility measures in patients with severe active rheumatoid arthritis
Measurement of health utility in rheumatoid arthritis
The Generic Health OMERACT rheumatoid arthritis study
Validity of EuroQol - A generic health status instrument in patients with rheumatoid arthritis
Measurement of the quality of life in rheumatic disorders using the EuroQol

Urology

Effectiveness and cost-effectiveness of TURP laser and waiting in the treatment of bladder outlet obstruction
An evaluation of a guideline-based open access urological investigation service
Assessment of alternative treatments for benign prostatic hyperplasia
Evaluation of treatments for patients with benign prostatic hyperplasia
Priontising a urological surgery waiting list

Others

Community-based leg ulcer clinics
Comparison of a variety of single index measures of quality of life in chronic illness
Electro-smog within the short-wave frequency range: Phantom or reality?
Estimating the burden of disease in The Netherlands
Evaluation of picture archiving and communication systems (PACS)
Impact of redundancy on health-related quality of life
QALY league tables for a hospital
Quality and cost-effectiveness of ambulatory medicine
Comparison of early discharge to hospital at home (HAH) scheme with continued hospital care
Solihull health outcomes priorities project

19
Not a quick fix

Martin Buxton

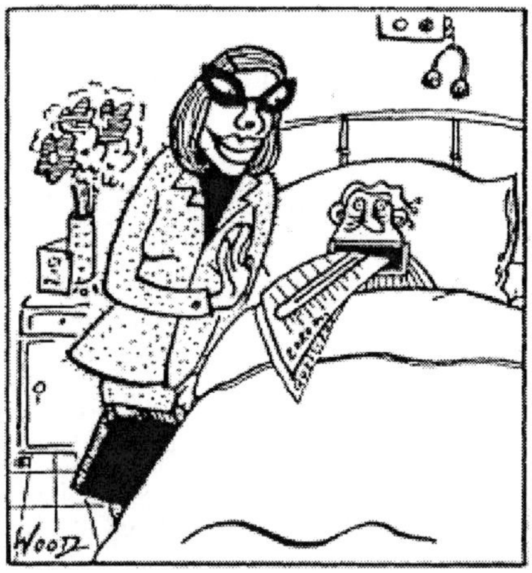

The EuroQol Group responds to criticism that its scheme for taking the 'temperature' of your health is a gimmicky solution to the problem of measuring outcomes

Roy Carr-Hill's recent warning against the use of the EuroQol system as a basis for decisions about allocating healthcare resources seems to be based on the fear that gullible managers will be tempted by the offer of a 'simple, quick solution to the problem of measuring outcomes' (Carr-Hill, 1991). As he says, it sounds too good to be true.

What puzzles us is where he got the impression that we are in the business of offering managers a quick fix. Our initial publication, to which his comments are mainly directed, made clear that the system was by no means in its final form and that the existing findings, derived from northern Europe, might not stand up if tested on populations with different cultural backgrounds (EuroQol Group, 1990).

We went on to invite researchers who were willing to help extend this work in a practical way to get in touch with us. Does this sound like promotion of a simple, quick solution to the problem of measuring outcomes? Moreover we explicitly stated that 'detailed work carried out during the development phase will be reported by individual researchers within the EuroQol Group', and some of it now has (and there is more to come) (Nord, 1991; Brooks *et al*, 1991; Essink-Bot *et al*, 1990).

P. Kind et al. (eds.), EQ-5D concepts and methods, 235–237.

Against that background let us examine Dr Carr-Hill's objections to our claim that the health state valuations elicited in our three initial surveys (in England, The Netherlands and Sweden) show remarkable similarity. Using conventional statistical tests we found strong support for our conclusions. All this is reported on page 206 of our article, though Dr Carr-Hill chooses to ignore it.

Instead he starts picking away at some selected differences between particular numbers in the table, and comes up with a list of 'quite large' differences in the valuations given (in all three countries) to being in no pain or discomfort as opposed to being in some pain or discomfort. But he is barking up the wrong tree here. What he needs to show is that the value attached to any particular change in health state is different between countries. This he fails to do. Indeed, had he pursued his method of analysis more systematically, he would have discovered that the 'quite large differences' simply evaporate.

His approach assumes that a worsening on one dimension is viewed in the same way, no matter what accompanies it. But we must keep open the possibility - supported by our data - that a worsening on one dimension (for example, pain and discomfort) is viewed one way if you are otherwise in good shape and another way if you are also somewhat immobile and unable to pursue your usual activities.

Only by working with composite states can we test whether where a person is on one dimension of health affects how they value a change in some other dimension. Dr Carr-Hill admonishes us for offering no justification for doing this, and warns that 'many authors have warned against this procedure', citing Froberg and Kane as authority, though we have failed to find any such warning in the source cited (Froberg and Kane, 1989). But even if we had, those authors would still have had to convince us that there is a better way of eliciting interactions.

Dr Carr-Hill also makes heavy weather of our use of a visual analogue scale in the form of a thermometer in order to elicit valuations from respondents. It was calibrated from zero to 100, and had ‘worst imaginable health state’ at the bottom, and 'best imaginable health state' at the top. From this he implies that we think the valuation of health states is like the measurement of heat. But social science data on values and opinions does not have to be like physical data before it can be useful. And we did not expect everyone to come up with the same valuations, or even the same rank orderings, and an important part of our research agenda is the systematic exploration of the relationships between valuations and the characteristics of respondents.

Finally let us turn to response rates, which we ourselves have described as 'rather disappointing' (Brooks *et al*, 1991). But whether they are, as Dr Carr-Hill claims, 'extraordinarily low when asking about health, even for a postal, self-completion questionnaire', remains to be demonstrated. To our knowledge no postal survey results have been published which attempted psychometric valuation of health states, as opposed to asking for fairly straightforward factual information.

We have obviously been trying to improve response rates, and a large survey by our Dutch colleagues, soon to be published, experimented with various response-influencing strategies. They have concluded that the highest response rate we could reasonably expect from a general population that is not specially motivated is around 60%, which still leaves us with some way to go, of course. But as we said in our original publication, 'there seems little danger of selection bias as valuations vary little with background variables or response times' (page 206). We are still working on this problem.

Constructive criticism is the purpose of publishing results in professional journals. Balanced comments from careful readers are always welcome, especially when they are directed towards helping the potential users of that work, in this instance hard-pressed health service personnel and policy makers. But busy and hard-pressed though they may be, we hope that readers of Dr Carr-Hill's comments and our reply to them will take time to read the original article and judge for themselves whether Dr Carr-Hill has in fact offered a balanced and constructive criticism based on a careful reading of the material.

Text prepared in response to Carr-Hill R. A good measure for Eurohealth?
Health Service J 1991;101:24-25

REFERENCES

Brooks R G, et al. EuroQol: Health-related quality of life measurement. Results of the Swedish questionnaire exercise. Health Policy 1991;18:37-48.

Carr-Hill R. A good measure for Eurohealth? Health Service J 1991;101:24-25.

Essink-Bot M L, et al. Valuation of health states by the general public: Feasibility of a standardised measurement procedure. Social Science and Medicine 1990;31:1201-1206.

EuroQol Group. EuroQol - A new facility for the measurement of health-related quality of life. Health Policy 1990;16:199-208.

Froberg D G, Kane R L. Methodology for measuring health state preferences I: measurement strategies. J Clinical Epidemiology 1989;42(4):345-54.

Nord E. EuroQol: health-related quality of life measurement. Valuations of health states by the general public in Norway. Health Policy 1991;18:25-36.

Postscript

Alan Williams

This second volume of papers emanating from the EuroQol Group should be seen not only as evidence of the scientific prowess of the contributors but also as a testimony to their personal qualities. For most participants active membership of the Group is both enjoyable and rewarding, but it is also quite stressful. The stress arises from several sources, not least of which is the heterogeneous nature of the Group. Anyone who has ever worked in a collegial (rather than a hierarchical) manner with strong-minded colleagues, even within the same discipline within the same country, will appreciate the high level of mutual respect and methodological tolerance that is called for if the enterprise is not to fall apart. When the Group consists of people drawn from different disciplines, with different research cultures, different methodological stances, seeking solutions that will work in very different institutional settings, and with careers of their own to pursue which in many cases attach higher prestige to work in your own mainstream discipline than to work undertaken with "outsiders", it is a minor miracle that the Group has not only survived for nearly 2 decades already, but also proved to be so productive both at a methodological and at a practical level.

A shared objective is, of course, a great help. From the outset the two principal objectives of the enterprise have distinguished it from most other researchers concerned with the measurement and valuation of health-related quality of life. Instead of trying to develop a measure that would comprehensively cover all attributes of that very wide-ranging concept, we sought instead to find a small "common core" of key attributes that most people regarded as the most important. Indeed, at the beginning we called ourselves "The Common Core Group". The second important objective was to move away from what the professionals regarded as the most important, and replace it with what the general public regarded as the most important. This was a major challenge, because most of the existing instruments were designed by professionals for the use of professionals in their own decision-making, so one of the principal criteria for choosing between instruments was their respective capacity to measure "clinically significant" changes. Our approach shifted the emphasis to testing how the changes in outcome that were brought about were valued by the people affected. This meant engaging in very complicated and expensive survey work amongst ordinary people as to how they valued different outcomes, and because we were so multinational (and became more so as new people came on board) this meant careful attention to translation and cross-cultural issues, a notoriously difficult field.

Generally speaking the Group itself has had only sparse resources of its own with which to commission work, and, especially at the outset, had to rely on each participating research group to raise its own money. So although we were able to identify research topics that needed tackling in order to further the Group's objectives, we

P. Kind et al. (eds.), EQ-5D concepts and methods, 239–240.

were utterly dependent on individuals volunteering to work on one or more of these, and to raise the money with which to do it. This raised delicate issues about intellectual property rights and about the sharing of data within the Group, all of which had to be negotiated within a collegial culture in which people's individual career prospects were often at stake.

Then, as the "common core" slowly crystallised and became what is now EQ-5D, we ran into further difficulties balancing the restless search for innovation and improvement against the need for some stability if we were to offer the outside world an instrument that did not change every year so that comparability with previously collected data was lost. Amongst the methodologists within the Group this was not too difficult a problem to solve in principle, because we adopted a rule that each experimental innovation must be evaluated against the status quo as the main comparator, so that we could see precisely what its impact would be. It was not sufficient to establish the theoretical superiority of a proposed change, we wanted to know its empirical significance too. But externally no such flexible convention was available so we had to bite the bullet and declare a moratorium on further variation in the instrument itself in order to provide a greater sense of security for users. The original idea was that after 3 or 4 years we would have accumulated enough well-tested improvements to produce a second version incorporating them all, taking as much care as we could to enable people to map the data from earlier version into the later one. In the event this proved to be much more difficult than we had expected, partly because of the tremendous ancillary investment that had been undertaken in producing versions of EQ-5D in many different languages (much of which would have to be redone), and partly because of the very heavy investment in valuations for the existing health states, which would also need revision. For the more radical innovators within the Group this remains a major source of frustration, since it leads to priority being given to revisions that can more readily be assimilated into the existing structure.

But what this all reflects are the tensions that are inherent in pioneering scientific work. Deep down you know that what you think you know is always contingent and contestable (even within the Group itself). So the best you can hope for is that enough of your colleagues will regard your (current) findings as a working hypothesis that they are willing accept until something better comes along. At a personal level the problem here is that if they are unwilling to do this, you may find it hard to resist taking it as a more personal rejection, and then the emotional level rises and interpersonal relationships are put under strain. Fortunately this has very rarely happened within the Group, which is why I observed at the outset that a rather special temperament is required of participants if they are to work productively within the peculiar ambience of the EuroQol Group. The old dictum about "No gain without pain" seems to sum it all up rather neatly.

CPSIA information can be obtained at www.ICGtesting.com
Printed in the USA
LVOW100227090312

272310LV00007B/8/P